THE
PMA
POSITIVE MENTAL ATTITUDE
METHOD

THE
PMA
— POSITIVE MENTAL ATTITUDE —
METHOD

14 DAYS **TO A STRONGER, HEALTHIER, HAPPIER YOU**

aster

FAISAL ABDALLA

An Hachette UK Company
www.hachette.co.uk

First published in Great Britain in 2018 by Aster,
a division of Octopus Publishing Group Ltd, Carmelite House,
50 Victoria Embankment, London EC4Y 0DZ
www.octopusbooks.co.uk
www.octopusbooksusa.com

Distributed in the US by Hachette Book Group, 1290 Avenue of the Americas,
4th and 5th Floors, New York, NY 10104

Distributed in Canada by Canadian Manda Group, 664 Annette St.,
Toronto, Ontario, Canada M6S 2C8

ISBN 978-1-91202-337-0

A CIP catalogue record for this book is available from the British Library.

Printed and bound in China.

1 3 5 7 9 10 8 6 4 2

All reasonable care has been taken in the preparation of this book, but the
information it contains is not meant to take the place of medical care under
the direct supervision of a doctor. Before making any changes in your health and
fitness regime, always consult a doctor. Any application of the ideas and information
contained in this book is at the reader's sole discretion and risk. Neither the author
nor the publisher will be responsible for any injury, loss, damages, actions,
proceedings, claims, demands, expenses and costs (including legal costs or expenses)
incurred in any way arising out of following the exercises in this book.

Contributing Editor Louise Abdalla

Consultant Publisher Kate Adams
Senior Designer Jaz Bahra
Senior Editor Leanne Bryan
Copy Editor Salima Hirani
Photographers Philip Haynes & Kris Kirkham
Food Stylist Becks Wilkinson
Prop Stylist Agathe Gits
Hair & Make-up Jo Adams & Jade Bird
Production Controller Beata Kibil

CONTENTS

PREFACE

I'm not going to thank you for buying my book, I'm going to applaud you. The chances are this is the start of your journey to a fit and healthy life, and that first step is always the scariest. Perhaps you've tried to change your life a few times before but, for whatever reason, it hasn't worked. That's okay. "Fear kills more dreams than failure ever will", as the saying goes. Don't be afraid of messing up along the way – we all do at some point.

You may have followed me for a while and want help maintaining your progress and staying on track. Whatever your reasons for reading this book, I've covered every angle so that, whatever your level, you will take something positive away from it. This book will help you to press the reset button and set you on the path towards a stronger, healthier, happier you. My 14-day training plan contains exercises to suit all abilities and, as you advance, the exercises will become more advanced too.

Starting and maintaining a health and fitness journey can be daunting, but it's not impossible. You need to challenge the negative thoughts telling you you're not good enough, strong enough, fast enough. All that matters is that you are brave enough. Be brave enough to take that first step towards being the best version of yourself and be brave enough to never look back.

You have just one life and it's not nearly long enough, so don't waste it being average. Set your sights higher and reach for what you deserve, not just for what's in easy reach. Tell yourself every day that you are not here to be average – you are here to be awesome.

Faisal

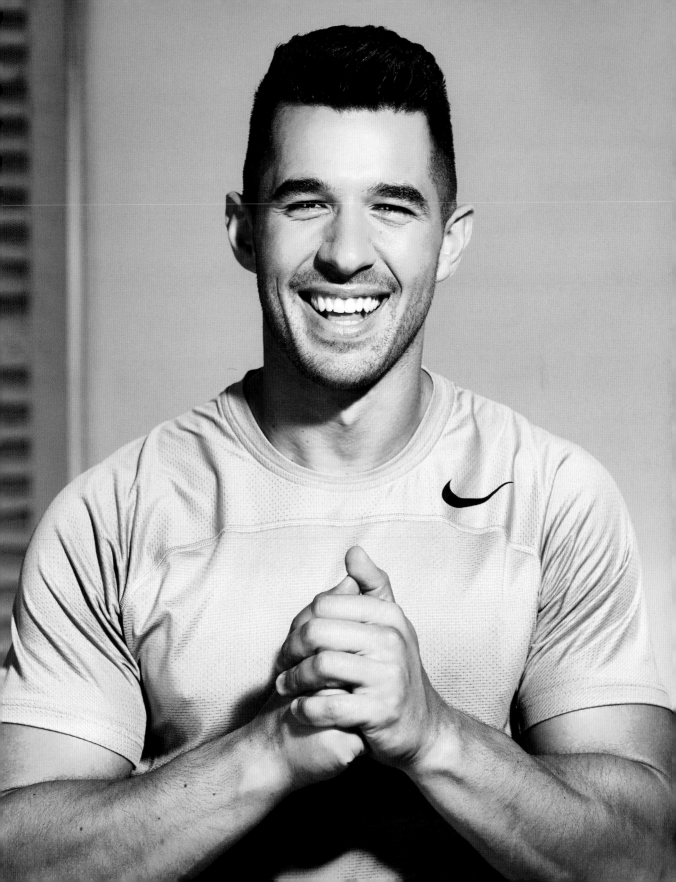

INTRODUCTION

Who is this very loud man with a quiff who is always banging on about PMA? Well, you are right to ask. I understand it may be hard to trust a man who smiles this much.

My name is Faisal and I'm a Nike Master Trainer (there are only a few of us in the UK – we're a protected species!). I'm also a Master Trainer at the fitness phenomenon Barry's Bootcamp, which specializes in sweaty, fast-paced HIIT workouts and attracts people from all walks of life. I'm perhaps best known for my work training celebrities such as full-time singer/part-time kickass ninja Ellie Goulding. And I pop up on your TV from time to time to encourage those of you at home to get moving. At some point between it all I try to get some sleep! I'm used to training people of all abilities, who have very different goals and do you know what? I love it, because it allows me to help people on their personal journeys and spread positivity while I do it.

MY FITNESS JOURNEY

I haven't always been a fitness trainer, but I have been interested in sports and fitness for as long as I can remember. I was a ball boy at Wimbledon, so I started on the right path, but then I moved on to do every job under the sun – I sold TVs, starred in music videos, twiddled my thumbs in an office, massaged people in nightclubs, I even played Postman Pat in pantomime! I was unfulfilled career-wise. I then became a struggling actor with dreams of making it in Hollywood and did a lot of extra work on movies such as *Inception, Edge of Tomorrow* and *Get Him to The Greek*. It was on film sets that my love of fitness really began and it sparked a passion that had been missing. On set, I used to hang

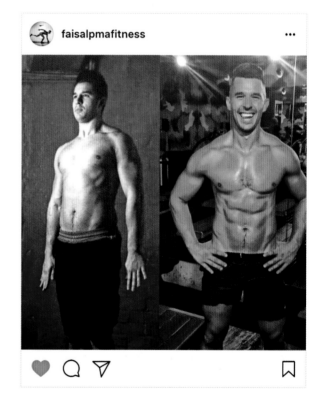

We were all beginners once (take a look at the picture on the left, compared to me, now, on the right). We all had to start somewhere, so don't feel intimidated. I understand what it is like to be on a journey because the journey never ends.

out with the stunt team between takes and became fascinated with strength and the human body. I began to train properly to see how far I could push my physical limits, which led me to this career.

Learning from experience

It took a long time for me to see real changes. I was putting in some serious hours at the gym but it wasn't quite paying off, as can be seen from the image opposite from my first ever fitness shoot in 2011. I wasn't performing at my best and, aesthetically, I wasn't the best version of myself. At the time I didn't know why. I was never massively overweight but, in my mid-twenties, when I should have been reaching my peak, I was still doing up my shoelaces at the bottom of the mountain. This was, I discovered, because I wasn't doing the right sort of training for me. That changed when I discovered high-intensity interval training (HIIT – see right).

When it came to nutrition, I didn't have a clue. I spent many dinners eating nothing but tuna from the can because I thought all I needed was protein, or I'd hit the drive-through after the gym, thinking I'd earned it. I would have a bag of sugar-laden caramel rice cakes in the car at all times and would eat an entire packet each day because I thought they were healthy. It's no wonder I wasn't seeing changes.

Slowly, it dawned on me just how important food was to my progression. The saying "you can't out-train a bad diet" couldn't be more true. I have worked hard to develop my training and hone my eating habits since then, and now I am truly happy with my body. This book puts right all the wrongs I was making back then so you don't waste time making the same mistakes.

I now tell people that success is down to 100 per cent training AND 100 per cent nutrition – I never said math was my strong point! The two go hand in hand and you need to give your full commitment to both if you want to succeed.

Fuss-free healthy diet

I feel it's important to say I'm not a nutritionist or dietician. I am also not a culinary wizard. I have, however, spent more than half my life training in a serious capacity and I am at the point where I'm confident I've found the right way to fuel my body to get the best results.

My approach to food is simple. I don't count macros (macronutrients – carbohydrates, fat and protein) or calories and I don't spend time weighing out my food – life is too short! I'm a man who loves his food, and I take a common-sense approach to it to maintain a healthy relationship with the food on my plate. To give my body the best-quality fuel, I try to choose healthy, fresh, additive-free ingredients, and find ways of making them taste good. It's that simple. I've discovered that eating well does not have to be boring, or require hours spent in the kitchen.

HIIT and strength training

My training method is a combination of high-intensity interval training (HIIT) and strength training. HIIT and its fat-burning benefits have absolutely transformed my body and fitness levels. Strength training works in perfect harmony with HIIT as it helps to sculpt and define lean muscle. If you want an all-round healthy body that's low in body fat, strong and physically fit when it comes to cardio, HIIT and strength training provide the perfect formula to help get you there.

Positive Mental Attitude

For me, the glue that holds everything together – the training and the healthy diet – is a positive mental attitude (PMA). I've been brought up with PMA, so it's not something I've massively struggled with. I've had hard times, when it has been tested, but luckily it has always held firm because it is engrained. I believe it is not what we go through that shapes us as a person, but how we choose to deal with it. In the words of the legend Rocky Balboa: "Nobody is gonna hit as hard as life. But it ain't about how hard you hit, it's about how hard you can get hit and keep moving forward".

I realized the importance of PMA when I started training clients. People would ask me how I was always smiling and so energetic. They'd ask for advice when they were struggling to stay motivated or for pep talks when they were held back by injury. Some were fed up because they felt they weren't progressing fast enough, while others would come to me for inspiration before a big race. I'd give advice and support to everyone, and soon learned that all roads led back to PMA – three simple letters that were simply life-changing if I could get people to understand their essence and really feel it in their hearts.

I suddenly understood more than ever the link between body and mind. Since then, I have worked tirelessly to spread the message of PMA, through motivational messages on social media and by trying to leave a positive impact on everybody I meet. That work has earned me the nickname Mr PMA, which seems to have stuck with everyone (except for my father-in-law, who thinks it's more amusing to call me Mr PMT). For anyone who wants to change their life for the better, I can think of no simpler way than to start with a positive mental attitude.

YOUR FITNESS JOURNEY STARTS NOW!

This is not just an exercise book and it is not merely a recipe book. It's about training your body *and* your mind. I want you to get mentally and emotionally fit in a way you have never done before.

The PMA Method

I'm half Egyptian so I love a pyramid (bear with me!). Imagine a pyramid with three sides – food, fitness and PMA (*see* right). That is what The PMA Method is all about. I believe you simply need to consistently think positively, eat well and get moving. It really doesn't need to get more complicated than that.

My aim is to teach you the basics of how I live and train so that you can do this whole being-fit-and-healthy thing on your own. Eventually, being healthy will change from something you are trying to do to somebody that you just are. Exercise and healthy eating can become second nature if you persevere and have fun along the way. Once you start to see results, you won't look back.

This method is not a quick fix or a crash diet. If you are thinking "What's the fastest way for me to lose weight?" then you need to rethink your approach and start looking at the long game. The aesthetic stuff comes naturally if you get yourself emotionally fit and make your health a priority, but you need to hustle for it. So stop looking for quick fixes and shortcuts because real changes that last you a lifetime are what you need.

The fuel

The messages around healthy eating can be confusing, with scientists and experts issuing different and often conflicting advice. But food should not be overwhelming – it should be something you enjoy.

People generally want to find a way of enjoying food that won't make them pile on pounds, that will help them define their bodies and give them all the energy and nutrients they need. This book offers an easy-to-follow approach that does just that, with a few tips on how to organize your food intake to maximize the benefits. Your social life doesn't have to end because you are on a strict diet. This is just good, tasty food to nurture body and soul.

The training

This is probably the hardest part. Exercise takes both time and commitment. You'll get sore, and there will be days when you'd rather clean the toilet than work out, but nothing worth having comes easy. Even now, I find it hard. I always say it never gets easier, you just get better.

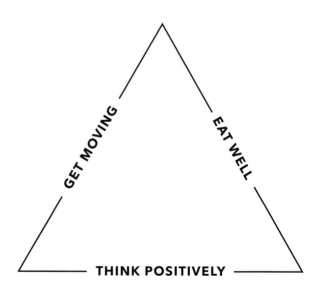

If you break it down, it really isn't that scary. These are three simple changes anyone can make, and the results can be huge, so go build that pyramid!

You can make it easier by not giving it 100 per cent and cheating on the timings if you want, but you are only cheating yourself. Honest training brings honest results. You will get out what you put in.

In chapter 4 of this book you will find HIIT workouts that focus on different areas of your body. This gives your muscles time to recover between sessions. You will also find each workout contains an element of strength training to help get your body stronger than ever. I also prescribe weekly rest/cheat days, because you are only human. For this to be sustainable, it needs to be livable.

The mindset

Once you learn the basics of what you should eat and how you should train, you're well on your way, and what will keep you on track is a positive mental attitude. So it's important to dedicate some energy to training the mind as well. It's your mind that holds all the power – the decision to either give up or power on comes from the mind. Once you've mastered the art of positive thinking, you will be a force to be reckoned with!

Follow my tips in the following chapter and stay positive every step of the way, even when that end goal seems like a tiny dot on the horizon. Learn to celebrate the small steps, and you will eventually make enough of them to get those big results.

Let's go!

So, there you have it – feeling fit and strong takes hard work and discipline, but it can and will be done. With The PMA Method, you can find the motivation to get on the right path and the commitment to stay on it.

If you open yourself to it, this book will help you to make the changes you need NOW. So, what are you waiting for? Forget "I'll start next week" and "On Monday I will start afresh". You might never run out of excuses, but one day you *will* run out of tomorrows, so make today the day you start kicking butt!

"I suffer from high-functioning anxiety, which has led to depression. I came across one of Faisal's Motivation Monday posts about being emotionally fit and it really spoke to me, and so I decided to look into what he meant by PMA. Faisal's constant good mood and motivational messages inspired me to try and do one small positive thing every day, and to take it step by step. I told myself that if he can be in a positive mood while fasting at 5am on the way to work, then I could also have the mental strength to get through situations I find testing that I try to avoid when my anxiety and depression are particularly bad. Faisal's posts remind me to try to have a positive outlook on a day-to-day basis. It has been refreshing to see a fitness influencer whose posts don't make me feel unhappy about my body not being perfect, or my mental health not being 100 per cent."

Anonymous, 28, London

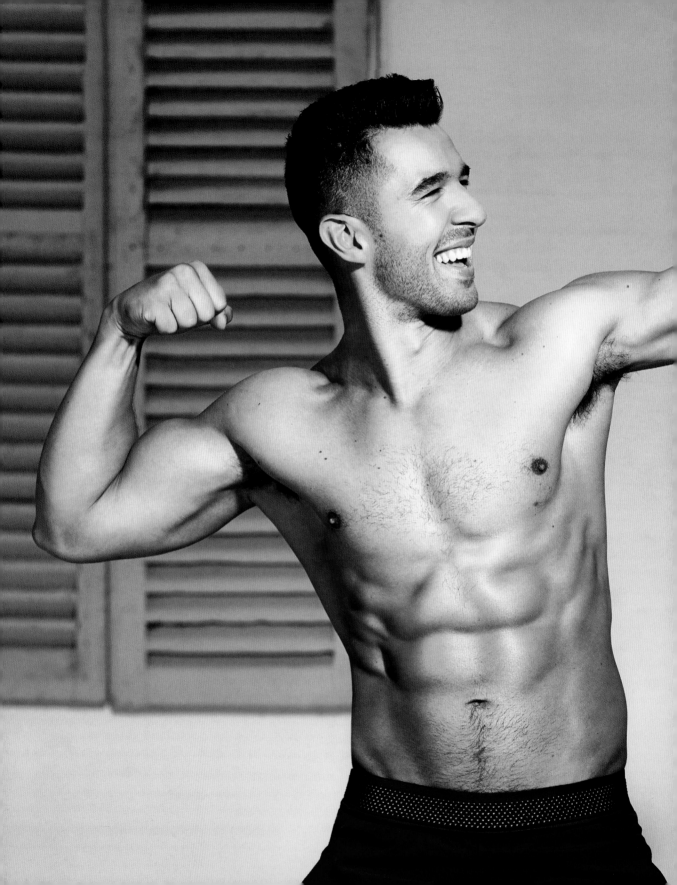

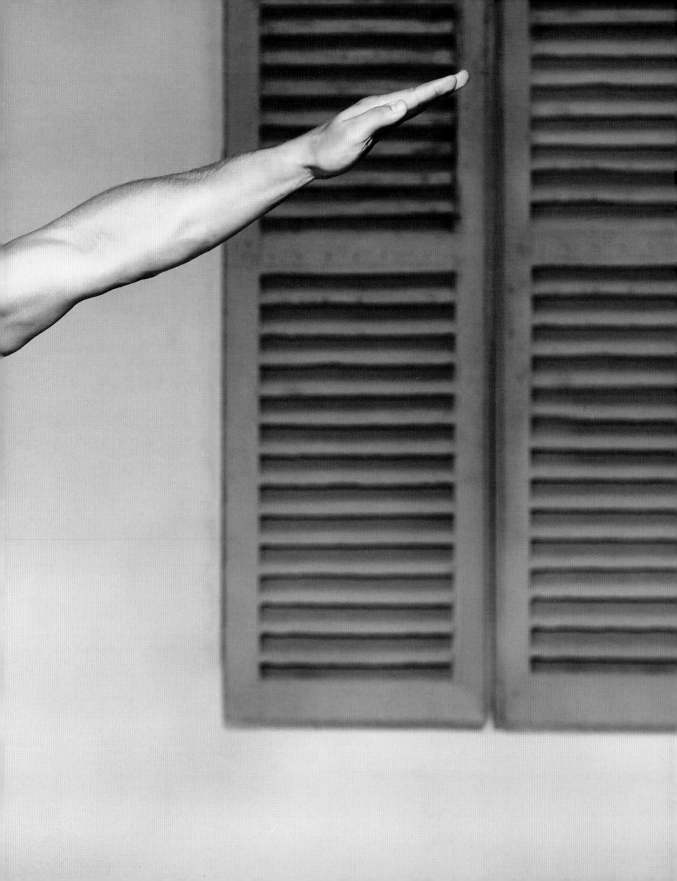

CHAPTER 1

PMA: THE MAGIC INGREDIENT

I know you guys love to learn new workouts and recipes, but it is vital that you get into the right headspace before you move on to any of that. Anyone can follow a workout or a recipe once, but the changes need to go deeper than that for them to last. It is PMA (positive mental attitude) that will help you continue to make good food choices when the novelty of healthy eating has worn off and you're craving a bucketload of fried chicken, or reach for the dumbbells when you'd rather veg out on the sofa in your pyjamas!

WHAT IS PMA?

PMA is a state of mind, a lifestyle, and the key to success. The best thing of all? It is absolutely free, because it's in your head. We all have it, we don't need to pay for it, we just need the tools to unlock it. PMA is looking for the positive in everything, it is seizing every opportunity, believing in yourself, challenging the negative voices, loving the life you've been given and HAVING FUN.

It's not your body that sets your limits, it's your mind. If your mind is constantly saying I can't, I won't, I shouldn't, then thank goodness you bought this book.

PMA is my mantra in life, it is like a religion to me and I swear by it, which is why I'm known as Mr PMA. My connection with the term began as an 11-year-old kid watching TV and eating cereal on the living room floor. It was back in 1996, when a washing powder advert starring sprinter Kriss Akabusi came onto the screen. He was trying to motivate a child before a school sack race by using Olympian Linford Christie as his inspiration. He told the kid, "If you want to perform like Linford, you've got to think like Linford. PMA". Suddenly the *Chariots of Fire* theme tune came on in the background as the kid jumped his way to victory. At that moment I decided I wanted to be a champion and PMA was going to get me there. I was a very impressionable child and it has stayed with me ever since.

The power of the mind

PMA can improve your life in every aspect imaginable, but in the world of health and fitness, PMA is an absolute game changer. Every person who has ever won gold in the Olympics or broken a world record believed it was possible with enough hard work. We are a product of our thoughts – what we think, we then become. I'm not saying we could all overtake Mo Farrah on the track, but we all have our personal goals, whether it be running a marathon, lifting our own body weight or mastering a headstand. We can only achieve it if we believe we can. Even if you don't hit your exact goal, you will be closer than if you had never even tried. For example, you may train to run a marathon in under four hours, but miss your goal on the day by a few minutes. The fact is, in having that goal in the first place you lapped every single person sat on the sofa and achieved something incredible.

How many times have you been close to giving up on a run, yet somehow got to the end? Or you've woken up on a Monday morning and thought, "I can't get through today" and, before you know it, it's Tuesday? That's not your body magically producing more energy or strength. That is the strength of your mind pulling you through. *That* is the power of PMA. Now, how much more could you achieve if you *actively* tried to harness this power?

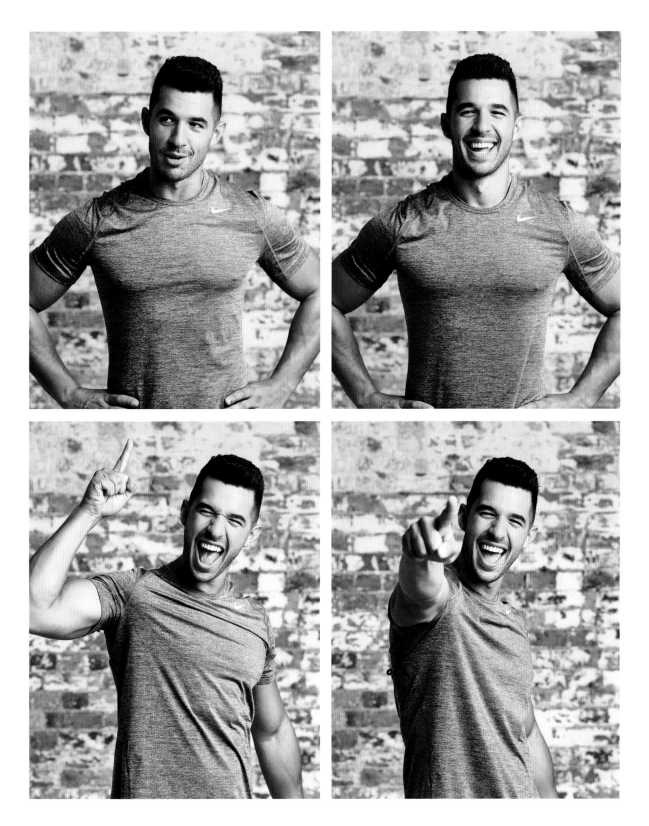

Break it down

It can help you psychologically to achieve your goals if you break them down into a series of mini-goals, then focus on these one at a time – and then celebrate each achievement. Want to eat better? Break it down – pay attention to a particular meal of the day, or master the art of meal preparation. Want to increase your core strength? Break it down – set yourself a plank challenge and add five seconds on each time. Keep going, keep pushing, and keep wanting more for yourself. Be realistic in your goals, but don't be afraid to be ambitious. It is okay to dream big and expect great things from yourself.

Celebrate the milestones

I have a pose that I throw up to celebrate whenever I hit a milestone, say, finishing a race, reaching a target, or training someone who has shown real grit or improvement. It isn't about flashing my biceps (although it's not bad for that!), it is a symbol of strength, success, empowerment and positivity. I have been doing it since I was a kid, after seeing an old photo of Arnold Schwarzenegger pulling the same pose. I also do it when I'm at an amazing viewpoint and loving the life I've been given, or whenever I feel grateful and believe that moment wouldn't have happened without PMA. For me, this pose has come to symbolize PMA and so has turned into something of a signature pose.

Amazingly, it has spread through my clients and followers who send me "PMA Postcards" showing them throwing up the pose all over the world (*see* opposite). I've had them from the Great Wall of China, Everest base camp, the Acropolis in Greece, the slopes of the Alps, Bali, Thailand, St Lucia, Italy... you name it! I've had air stewardesses, a 70-year-old woman and even newborn babies doing the pose (with a little help from Mum!).

TESTIMONIALS

PMA is a life-changing state of mind. I have had cards from people who say PMA has given them the courage to leave their jobs and pursue their dreams. One guy from Florida who had never run seriously in his life entered a marathon after watching my Motivation Monday videos. Even more powerful was a message I received from a young lady who had been suicidal and said my positivity helped her turn her life around. Scattered through the book are some testimonials from my clients and online followers. I've seen time and time again that it's not just me who benefits enormously from PMA. You can, too.

"When I first met Faisal I wondered, why is this dude banging on about PMA? The cynical side of me questioned whether it was just words which sounded good. But, fast-forward to just a couple of sessions later and I was hooked. Since I have started training with Mr PMA my outlook has shifted from being bronze-level positive to platinum status. I am 100 per cent more body confident, not only because I am physically stronger, but because he lifts you to new heights on a mental level where you believe you can achieve anything you work for."

Lynne Counsell, 39, London

"For me, as I got older, it became harder to motivate myself to get to the gym. Faisal has completely changed that. His positive mental attitude may be a catchphrase, but it actually works. He is the driving force behind me pushing myself to my absolute limits. His positive energy makes such a massive difference and, what is very clear, he genuinely does care about helping everyone achieve their very best."

Joe Heraty, 36, London

The photographs of PMA poses opposite have been sent to me from all around the world. Can you top them? Upload yours to Instagram and @faisalpmafitness along with #PMAPose.

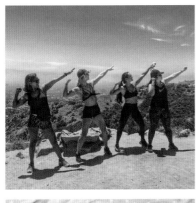 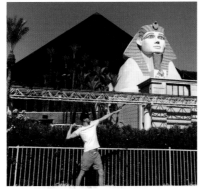 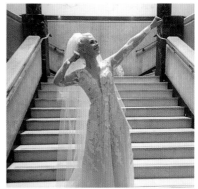
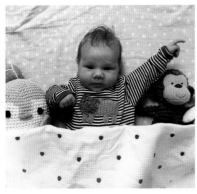 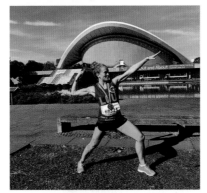 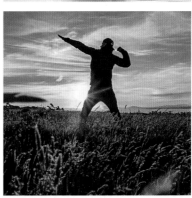
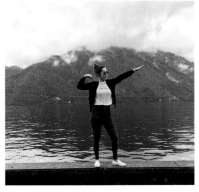 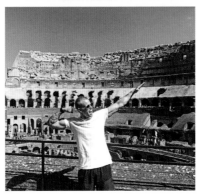 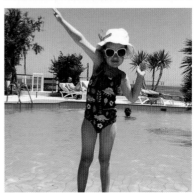
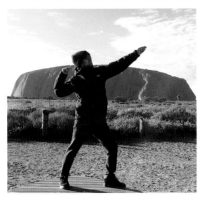 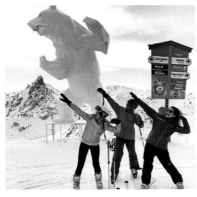 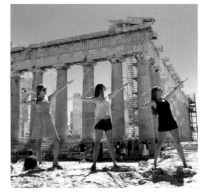

10 WAYS TO UNLOCK YOUR PMA

Below, I offer you my techniques for keeping a positive mental attitude at even the most testing of times. There's nothing complicated about PMA. What's hard is changing mental habits. To learn new skills, you have to train the mind just as you would the body, so return to this section and read the following guidelines again whenever you feel negative, to help you get back on track with your mental and emotional fitness.

1. ACTIVELY SEEK OUT THE POSITIVES

It's natural for bad things to happen in life, but there is *always* a positive in every situation - look for that positive. If you begin each day with a positive mindset, you will be more open to seeing the good in situations, so start each day with a positive affirmation (*see* page 20 for some tips). Repeat your affirmation out loud a few times and, if you want, write it down, screenshot it on your phone and look at it throughout the day.

2. CHALLENGE NEGATIVE THOUGHTS

It is your mind that first tells you, "No" when your legs are shaking from a torturous round of squats. But when training starts to hurt, it starts to work, so it's important to battle through the pain - unless you're injured, of course. It is your mind that tells you to eat a cookie before your hand physically reaches for the biscuit tin, so there is always time to do the right thing if you can challenge the negative thought in time.

Find a technique that works for you. For instance, when you are training and feel like quitting, sing something like "I can, I can, I can" in your head to your favourite tune to push the negativity out of your mind. Or decide on a "reserve" that you must tap into before you are allowed to stop. This could be two more reps, or 10 extra seconds of running, but whatever it is, you MUST stick to it. Talk to yourself, tell yourself you are strong enough, then finish the task with an empty tank knowing you gave it everything.

3. STOP COMPARING YOURSELF TO OTHERS; THEY AREN'T YOU!

We have a bad habit of only comparing ourselves to people who we think are better than us, which can make us feel inadequate. Everybody has their own strengths and goals, so focus on yourself and what you want to achieve. I train people to be the best they can be, not the best, full stop. Work on yourself, for yourself - you are your only competition.

Every time you find yourself comparing yourself to others in the gym or on social media in a way that makes you feel bad about yourself, give yourself a tap on your hand. This might sound crazy, but it snaps you out of the thought process and makes you aware that you are slipping into a bad place.

4. WHAT IS YOUR WHY?

Your *why* runs far deeper than your goals. You might want to lose a few pounds, tone your abs or be fit enough to run a marathon, but *why*? Perhaps you want to be a positive role model for your family, you want to address your mental health issues, or you want to live as long as possible to watch your children grow. Identifying your why can be hard and can force you to look at things you prefer to block out. But once you understand your why, you can visualize it when feeling unmotivated. It is one of the most powerful tools you have, so when you're disheartened with training, or want to bury your head in chocolate cake, remember *why* you want this.

5. DON'T BE TOO HARD ON YOURSELF

While it is great to have an end goal, don't be so blinded by how far you've got to go that you can't see how far you've come. Keep a training diary (*see* pages 38-9) so you have something to feel proud of. Celebrate the small steps as much as the giant leaps because they add up. See them as a milestone on your journey.

6. BE REALISTIC

It takes a good two or three months to really see changes, so do not give up when you don't drop a dress size overnight or, after a week of sit ups, a six pack hasn't magically appeared.

Remember, also, that you're only human and you're on a new journey, so if you take a wrong turn or fall off the wagon, don't use that as an excuse to give up. You're still breathing, so pick yourself up, get a grip and get back on the wagon - it takes far less energy than beating yourself up over a bar of chocolate that cannot uneat itself! Setbacks will happen - prepare for them so you can take them in your stride.

7. CHOOSE POSITIVE PEOPLE

Drop those around you who punctuate their sentences with "can't", "won't" and "don't". Surround yourself with positive friends - they will lift you higher, support your journey and keep you on track. If you feel that someone is toxic, you should reconsider their place in your life. If the cons outweigh the pros in a friendship, then what are you doing? Stop wasting your life and risking your happiness by clinging on to relationships that aren't good for you.

8. HAVE FUN!

If you aren't having fun and enjoying exercise then you haven't found the right training for you. That's fine. Move on and try something new, just don't quit. Try recruiting a friend, making an awesome workout playlist, changing the time you work out or taking your training outdoors to see if that makes a difference. Being healthy and working out should be a pleasure, not a chore, if you want to stick with it. So be flexible and play with the formula until you find what works for you.

9. BE GRATEFUL

Thankfulness is a powerful art you need to master. They say it's not happy people who are thankful, but thankful people who are happy. Take a second to fully appreciate the good times and ensure you don't let beautiful moments pass you by without fully appreciating them. Throwing up my PMA pose (*see* page 17) is a great way to acknowledge how grateful you are at any given moment.

10. TAKE OWNERSHIP

You are the one who needs to put the training work in, *you* are the one who needs to stick to eating well and *you* are the one who needs to stay positive and believe in yourself. Only you know if you are truly giving it your all, so be honest with yourself, take responsibility for yourself and own it, because it's not going to own itself.

GET STARTED!

Just starting is often the hardest part, but don't waste your life waiting for tomorrow. How many Mondays have been and gone where you've said I will start next week? The time is NOW. Join a gym, go for a walk, throw out your chocolate, do a home workout video, take the stairs - whatever the first step is, don't wait until tomorrow to take it. The new you starts right now, this second.

"After years of unsuccessfully dabbling with fitness and healthy diet I discovered Faisal and everything he stands for... PMA! From that point on I thought 'this is for me'. I'm now four stone down and part of a team teaching clubbercise and zumba classes. A half marathon and various charity races later, I am in better shape and happier than I have ever been. I feel at least 20 years younger. Faisal helped change my life. PMA is the best."

Suzy Hildreth, 42, West Midlands

POSITIVE AFFIRMATIONS

Affirmations are positive statements you repeat which help you overcome negative thoughts and replace them with positive ones. With enough repetition, they sink into your subconscious and become your reality. Look on the internet to find affirmations that suit you, or make up your own. Bear in mind the following pointers.

SAY YOUR AFFIRMATIONS OUT LOUD

This will help reinforce the words and increase their power. Saying them in front of the mirror can have an even greater affect.

MAKE THEM IN THE PRESENT TENSE

Use phrases that start with "I am", "I have" and "I do" rather than "I will", "I could", "I'm going to". Your words will have more impact if you are committing to them in the here and now.

GET COMFORTABLE WITH BEING UNCOMFORTABLE

If your affirmation makes you cringe, your discomfort might be because the words touch on a subject that makes you uncomfortable and therefore needs your attention. In which case, you need to repeat that affirmation even more to turn it into reality.

MAKE THEM REALISTIC

Don't say you have the perfect body if you don't believe you do because you will feel like you are repeating a lie. Be honest, with something like, "I want to lose my beer belly and I am confident that I can. I am a determined person and I can do this".

DON'T USE AFFIRMATIONS THAT CONTAIN NEGATIVE WORDS

Avoid words such as "can't" or "won't", because your mind will have to work harder to turn them into positives. For example, instead of saying, "I won't be stressed" try, "I am calm. I can control this situation".

Your mind is a creature of habit. Saying affirmations will feel awkward and alien at first, but it will soon come naturally and you won't even think about it. It takes a minimum of 21 days to create a new habit, and that includes positive thinking, so stick with it.

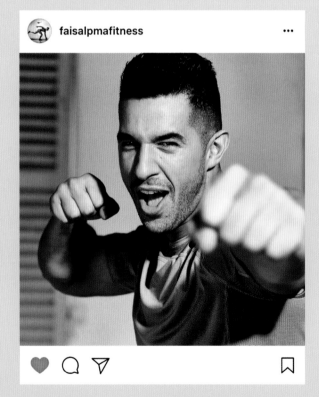

faisalpmafitness

MY FAVOURITE MOTIVATIONAL MANTRAS

"HONEST TRAINING, HONEST RESULTS"

"HEALTH IS WEALTH"

"DON'T LIMIT YOUR CHALLENGES. CHALLENGE YOUR LIMITS"

"BE THE BEST VERSION OF YOU"

"NOTHING WORTH HAVING COMES EASY"

"WHEN IT STARTS TO HURT, IT STARTS TO WORK"

"LOOK IN THE MIRROR; THAT'S YOUR COMPETITION"

"WHAT IS YOUR WHY?"

"IT DOESN'T GET EASIER, BUT YOU GET BETTER"

"GET COMFORTABLE WITH BEING UNCOMFORTABLE"

"LIFE BEGINS AT THE END OF YOUR COMFORT ZONE"

"DON'T BE AFRAID OF YOUR WEAKNESSES. LOOK THEM IN THE EYE AND TURN THEM INTO STRENGTHS"

"EAT, SLEEP, PMA, TRAIN, REPEAT"

"WHY BE AVERAGE WHEN YOU CAN BE AWESOME?"

CHAPTER 2

FUEL YOUR FITNESS

When it comes to eating well, there's a lot of information out there – we have fasting, juicing, counting macros, cabbage soup plans, fairy-dust diets – you name it! If they work for you and make you happy, great! But I think healthy eating should be simpler. As a man who is fond of his food and needs good fuel for an active life, I've put much energy into getting my diet just right. And guess what? I've discovered that healthy eating is achievable, sustainable and very enjoyable.

GOOD FUEL

I passionately believe that food should be something you enjoy. You just need to find a way of enjoying it that allows you to stay healthy. We are pretty useless engines without the right fuel. In order to achieve your physical goals, it's important to feed your body the right things – it's that simple.

My recipes are full of "good" carbs, "good" proteins and "good" fats (*see* table, page 24), with plenty of fresh vegetables and fruit.

Carbohydrates

Shock! Horror! Carbs are not the devil! The emphasis should be on *when* you eat them. When you train, you dip into your carbohydrate stores for energy (glycogen, if you want the jargon). We need to top up those stores after training so we have them sat there, ready for the next session. If the carb levels run low when exercising, the body thinks, "Damn I'm tired, what else can I burn for energy?" We don't want to eat into those muscles we have worked so hard to sculpt, so it's important we don't skip our carbs post-workout.

If we eat carbs and don't train, our full carbohydrate (glycogen) stores have nowhere to go. So our fat stores open their doors and say, "Hey buddy, come and stay here". To avoid storing our carbohydrates as fat, we need to keep that door shut! Therefore, if we are not training enough to dip into those glycogen stores and deplete them, we don't need a big old dose of carbs to top them up. For that reason, I eat good carbs post-training, and ensure other meals are low in carbs. With this in mind, the bulk of my recipes have been designed to be low-carb, with a carbohydrate "pimp it up post-workout" option for post-training meals.

Check out the table on page 24, which outlines the carb goodies. You will see that fruit and veg are on the list. Yes, they contain carbs, but they are also packed with vital vitamins and nutrients, and our bodies need this goodness to thrive. We will just try to concentrate on the lower-carb fruit and veg for your low-carb meals and save the higher-carb fruit and veg for post-training meals. As for the carb baddies, such as those you find in fizzy drinks, cookies and sweets, check out the table on page 24. We will be avoiding those!

Proteins

We also need protein after a workout because it helps muscle synthesis – another bit of jargon, but it basically

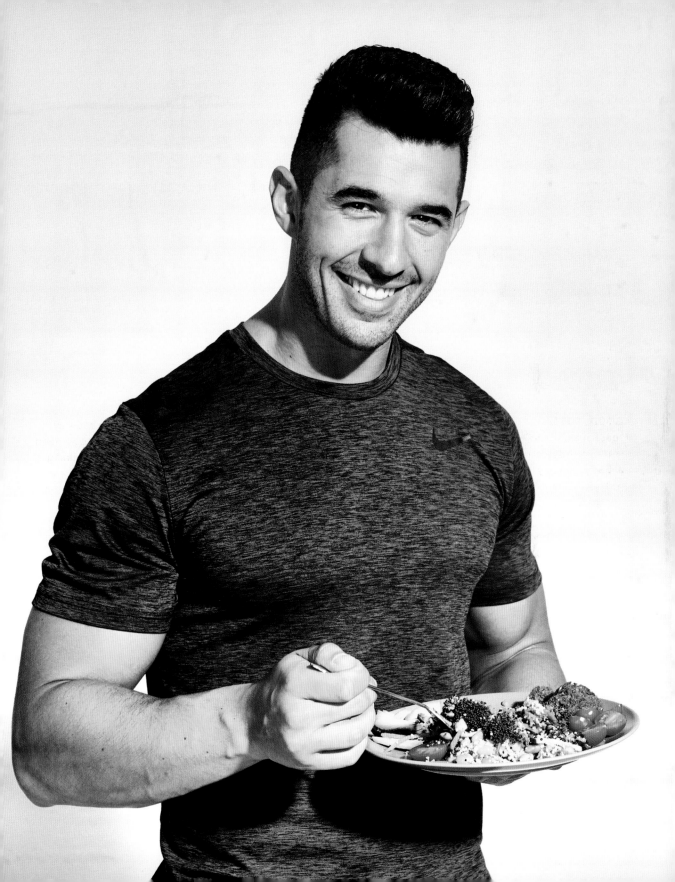

means we need protein to help our muscles grow and repair after exercise. Protein is a food source I recommend you eat with every meal if you can, not just after a workout. Whether you're looking to build muscle, lose weight, do both or maintain your current state, protein will help. Animal and plant proteins also help improve brain function, stabilize blood sugar levels and provide some of the building blocks of healthy bones. Check out the table below for a list of good proteins to build your meals around.

Fats

Just the word "fat" itself has negative connotations, so people fear it – they think that if they eat fat, they get fat.

GOOD CARBS	GOOD PROTEINS	GOOD FATS	CARBS TO AVOID
HIGHER-CARB FOODS (limit consumption to post-training)	Poultry – chicken, turkey	Avocado	Refined carbohydrates (forms of sugars and starch that don't exist in nature)
Oats	Cottage cheese	Whole eggs (don't bin that yolk)	White bread
Grains – barley, rye, buckwheat	Quark	Nut and seed butter (read labels and ensure there's no added sugar)	White pasta
Brown/wholegrain rice	Eggs		White rice
Quinoa	Full-fat milk	Oils – extra virgin olive oil, sesame oil, flax oil, coconut oil, avocado oil	White wraps
Beans, lentils, peas	Meat – lean lamb, beef and pork		White bagels
Wholemeal bread	Soya – soya milk, tofu, tempeh	Seeds – pumpkin, sesame, sunflower, flaxseed	Muffins
Wholemeal pasta	Fish and seafood		Sugary energy/cereal bars
High-carb (starchy) veg – potato, sweet potato, parsnip, sweetcorn, butternut squash, celeriac	Beans and pulses	Olives	Sweets
High-carb fruits – apple, banana, grape, pear, pineapple, figs		Oily fish – salmon, mackerel, anchovies, sardines and herring	Milk and white chocolate
		Nuts – walnuts, Brazil nuts, hazelnuts	Biscuits and cookies
LOWER-CARB FOODS			Fizzy drinks
Low-carb veg – cauliflower, cabbage, aubergine, green beans, asparagus, celery, mushrooms, peppers, courgette, radish, cucumber, onion			Ice cream
Leafy greens – kale, watercress, spring greens, chard			High-sugar cereals
Salad greens – romaine, chicory, spinach			Ketchup and other sugary sauces
Low-carb fruits – watermelon, melon, strawberry, raspberry, peach, blackberry, apricot			Alcohol

But the truth is that we need good fats in our diet for fuel and for the absorption of vital nutrients. There are different types of fat, and saturated and unsaturated fats such as monounsaturates and polyunsaturates are the ones we need (in moderation). The baddies are trans fats – the artificial hydrogenated nasties. We will be giving those a miss.

SMART FOOD SWAPS

AVOID	HEALTHIER SUBSTITUTE
Fruit juice	Real fruit
Milk and white chocolate	Dark chocolate
Sugary cereal	Porridge or overnight oats
White bread	Wholegrain or rye bread
Fizzy cola	Water or some fresh fruit juice with soda water
Salted nuts	Plain or home-roasted nuts
Sugar	Raw honey, maple syrup, ground sweet cinnamon, vanilla extract
Pizza	Homemade pizza on wholemeal pitta (see page 207)
White rice	Brown rice or cauliflower rice (see pages 188-9)
Low-fat strawberry yogurt	Plain Greek yogurt blended with fresh strawberries (see page 131)
Mayonnaise	Mashed avocado
White spaghetti	Wholemeal spaghetti or courgetti (see page 193)
Couscous	Quinoa
Crisps	Oven-roasted kale chips (see pages 178-9)
Dried fruit	Fresh fruit
Sugary energy/cereal bar	Handful of nuts
Ice cream	Blended frozen banana

"I have been training with Faisal for three years. There are very few things that have kept my interest and enthusiasm in London for as long. The simple truth is that his approach and techniques work. It's not just the exercises, it's the fact that he makes me want to do them, to improve myself, to be my best. He notices progress and celebrates it. Faisal's approach leaves me feeling better about myself and my place in the world."

Richard Cook, 45, London

"After following Faisal on social media, his contagious PMA motivated me to start setting new fitness goals for myself and inspired me to run my first marathon! Applying his PMA approach and mindset to everything I do has helped me achieve consistent improvements in both my fitness and all other aspects of life."

Jacob Noel Gonzalez, 24, Orlando, FL USA

THE FOOD PLAN

Now that you know what to eat, let's get you started! Healthy eating is all about simple, tasty food you can eat around your training. I have spent over half my life training in a serious capacity. I've tried and failed more times than I can remember, but I've finally found a way to eat that perfectly complements my training and helps me to squeeze out absolutely everything I can from every single workout.

I eat "farm to fork" whenever possible – fresh food, that has been through minimal processing. If I don't recognize an ingredient listed on the packet, I tend to avoid the product and find a fresher alternative. Food is not just calories, it's information that makes your body do what you want it to. We need to ask ourselves with every food choice, "What will this food do for me?"

Sugar does very little for you. It is addictive, it causes massive energy slumps and can cause you to overeat because it leaves you hungry. Most of us can identify the obviously sugary stuff – alcohol, fizzy drinks, cakes, biscuits and chocolate – but there are hidden sugars in many foods, such as mayonnaise, energy bars, ketchup and fruit juices. And there are many different names for sugar, making it difficult to avoid. The key is learning to check labels and spot sugar in its many guises. Avoid added and refined sugar until your cheat day (see below).

If you need something sweet in a recipe, use raw honey, maple syrup, dates, sweet cinnamon, mashed bananas or vanilla extract. Pure maple syrup and raw honey are very sweet, so a little goes a long way and, unlike refined sugar, they have some nutritional benefits. But don't fall into the trap of drowning everything in honey because you think it is good for you. It still contains sugar, so approach with caution!

#CheatDay

And for your diet to work in the long term, it must be sustainable and realistic. It is mentally draining to permanently deny yourself all your favourite foods, making it easy to slip back into bad habits that way.

I stay on track with a cheat day every Sunday. That way, I never feel as though I'm going without, and I don't veer off course during the week because I know there's a cheat day coming soon. I also take my day off from training on my cheat day, so I can spend the day relaxing and enjoying a treat or two with zero guilt – which helps to keep that PMA in good shape, too! (After all, this is a life-long commitment, and I'd rather not face a lifetime without Peanut M&M's, thank you very much.) Come Monday, I'm primed and ready to get back to the hard graft for another six days. Do be sensible and maybe look at it as a cheat meal instead of an entire 24 hours of bingeing! And, remember – honest training equals honest results. If you haven't trained as hard as you should have done during the week, be honest with yourself and skip the cheat day.

Make it sustainable

In my recipes (see pages 128–217), I've kept sustainability in mind. The dishes are quick and easy to make. And I go for no-fuss ingredients. Baobab, maca, lucuma, acai, goji, yuzu, pickled mountain ox tusk activated in unicorn juice… don't expect these in my recipes. Food doesn't have to contain expensive, fashionable ingredients and the latest superfoods to be healthy. Don't be put off by long ingredients lists – the ingredients are usually thrown into a bag together to marinate, or whacked into a food processor and chopped together.

Carb options

As I mentioned, each of my recipes offers easy post-workout options for you to pimp them up if you are eating to refuel after you train. We all train at different times, so I have provided post-workout options for each meal, to work around your schedule. If you haven't trained, make the meals without the carb options. If you have trained up to an hour and a half before eating, go for the post-workout option. Simple.

If in doubt, remember this formula:

"GO HARD = EAT CARBS AT REST = GIVE CARBS A REST"

Vegetarian options

I include many vegetarian recipes, which appear with a #MeatfreeMonday tag, as do the vegetarian alternatives for meat and fish dishes. I enjoy a Meatfree Monday once a week to give my body a little detox after my cheat day. Cutting down on my meat consumption one day a week is also my small gesture towards helping the environment and I encourage everybody to try it.

#FaisalFakeaway

As well as my beloved cheat days, I eat "fakeaways" when I crave a naughty takeaway. They are healthier versions of some of my favourite takeaway foods and are life-savers when I fancy a cheeky curry on a Friday night. They taste as good as takeaways but have an extra portion of nutrition and zero helpings of regret. Be sure to look out for the #FaisalFakeaway banner when you flick through the recipes.

When to eat

If you want to see serious changes from regular training, you need to fuel your body, not starve it. Going into starvation mode is massively counterproductive because your poor hungry body will try to retain calories in the form of fat cells. Bad news for weight loss. As a general rule, you should be looking to eat breakfast, lunch, dinner and, if you really need them, an absolute maximum of two small snacks each day. Do not skip your meals.

Eating pre-workout

If you are eating correctly throughout the day, you should not need to eat just because you are about to work out. This is a common trap that people fall into. They think they should eat before a workout for energy, then refuel right after, so they end up consuming more calories than they burn without realizing.

I drink branched-chain amino acids (BCAAs) mixed with water before a workout. These are great for muscle repair, so if you're doing multiple workouts in a week your muscles recover faster and ache less. They also prevent fatigue if drunk during training. If you want to give them a go, look for a 2:1:1 ratio when purchasing.

However, please listen to your body. If you are starving and have zero energy, eat something light such as an

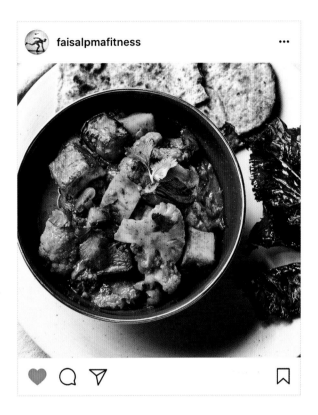

faisalpmafitness

apple, pear or 2–3 medjool dates with a tablespoon of nut butter. Or you could eat one of my Bounty Sea Salt Bombs (see page 210) for a quick energy hit. Try to eat it about half an hour before training to avoid stitch. There are no hard-and-fast rules here, apart from the fact that your health and wellbeing are number one.

Eating post-workout

Think of your muscles as a sponge post-workout. What you feed them right after training is important, as that's when the muscles are primed to absorb the nutrients they need to recover. Exercise breaks down muscle proteins, so protein post-workout is essential for repairing those muscle proteins and building new muscle tissue. And you need carbs to restore glycogen stores post-workout, too. Proteins and carbs work best together, so combine them in a meal. Just don't overload on the carbs – they should fill only a quarter of your plate.

MY KITCHEN TIPS

Cooking is time consuming and many of us would rather be eating food than making it. I look at time in the kitchen with a business mind and ask myself, what's the most time-efficient way to do this? Here are some helpful tips to reduce the time you spend chained to the cooker.

PLAN AHEAD

Plan your meals at the start of the week so you have the right ingredients in the house. This will help you to prepare in advance and organize your food around your training.

BATCH-COOK AND FREEZE

I am very pro batch-cooking – my motto is cook once, eat twice. When I cook I make more than I need and freeze the extra portions, so I always have meals available if I'm short of time. I also use the freezer to store leftovers and bread. Freezer bags are great for this because they take up less space than plastic containers.

ICE CUBE TRAYS ARE AWESOME

They help you cut down on food waste and massively reduce food prep. You can freeze homemade pesto, fresh herbs in olive oil, grated ginger, puréed garlic, chopped chilli, lemon juice – you name it.

INVEST IN A BLENDER

You can spend a lot on a blender, but there are cheaper versions out there that do the trick. Blenders shave so much time off your cooking. I use mine for the obvious things like smoothies and soups, but they are also great for making dressings and sauces. If you cannot be bothered to chop, just whack it all in and whiz it up.

KEEP CUPBOARDS STOCKED

I ensure I always have the basics in the cupboard so I can make a no-fuss meal if the refrigerator is empty. If I have herbs, spices, chickpeas, lentils, tuna, nuts, seeds, passata, brown rice, quinoa, chopped tomatoes and oils, I can normally rustle up something good.

STOCK THE HERB SHELF

I prefer to use fresh herbs, but they spoil quickly, so I keep my dried herb shelf well stocked. A good rule is to use 1 teaspoon of dried herbs in place of 1 tablespoon of fresh. Herbs add bags of flavour to simple, healthy food.

PRE-MIX FAVOURITE SPICE BLENDS

If you cook certain meals a lot, pre-mix your spices in large batches to save yourself time when you cook. I save empty jars, fill them with pre-mixed herb and spice blends and label them.

KEY PRINCIPLES FOR HEALTHY EATING

FUEL YOUR BODY, DON'T STARVE IT. EAT THREE HEARTY MEALS A DAY, PLUS A MAXIMUM OF TWO SNACKS, IF NEEDED.

DON'T EAT JUST BECAUSE YOU ARE ABOUT TO WORK OUT. IF YOU'RE STARVING AND HAVE NO ENERGY, HAVE A LIGHT SNACK HALF AN HOUR BEFORE YOU TRAIN.

DRINK BCAA POWDER WITH WATER BEFORE TRAINING TO BOOST ENERGY AND AID POST-WORKOUT RECOVERY.

TRY TO REFUEL WITHIN THE "GOLDEN HOUR" POST-WORKOUT.

SAVE THE CARBS FOR POST-WORKOUT MEALS AND EAT THESE ALONG WITH PROTEIN.

INCLUDE SOME PROTEIN AND A SMALL AMOUNT OF GOOD FAT IN ALL OTHER MEALS AS WELL AS SOME LOW-CARB FRUIT AND VEG.

BATCH-COOK, PRE-MIX SPICES AND GET AHEAD TO SAVE TIME AND PREVENT SLIP-UPS.

TREAT YOURSELF TO A WEEKLY CHEAT DAY AND SUBSTITUTE #FAISALFAKEAWAYS FOR TAKEAWAYS.

FOCUS ON NUTRIENTS RATHER THAN MACROS OR CALORIES.

AVOID REFINED AND ADDED SUGARS; EAT UNPROCESSED FOOD AND ADOPT A "FARM TO FORK" APPROACH.

STAY HYDRATED; H_2O IS ESSENTIAL FOR METABOLISM, MUSCLE REPAIR AND MORE.

CHAPTER 3

TRAIN WITH ME

When I discovered high intensity interval training (HIIT), my body really began to change – my body fat went down, my definition increased, my cardio performance drastically improved and I started to feel really energized. I recommend HIIT to everyone as part of a weekly workout routine. It is hugely effective in a short amount of time and you can do it almost anywhere.

Years of experimenting have shown me that the best way for me and my clients to train is to use a combination of zonal HIIT and strength-based training. This combination will help you to effectively burn fat and build muscle at a steady rate.

What is HIIT?

HIIT consists of short periods of all-out, quick, intense exercise to get the heart rate up, followed by short periods of rest or active recovery. Interval training is one of the most time-efficient ways to train. It is great for burning calories (which continues even after exercising), boosts your metabolism, increases endurance, torches fat and is great for heart health.

What is strength training?

Strength training means using a resisting force, such as dumbbells or resistance bands, to exercise muscles in order to build their strength. It is about so much more than bulking up – being strong is incredibly empowering and helps you in ways that go far deeper than surface aesthetics. It improves joint function and mobility, and is a massive contributor to overall health and wellness. It is also a great fat burner – the more muscle mass you have, the higher your metabolic rate, which means the more calories you burn, even at rest.

In this book, you will find lots of tempo strength training exercises using body weight or dumbbells. Tempo training means slowed-down exercises using weights. Rather than smashing out as many bicep curls as possible, I will occasionally encourage you to slow down the moves, which gives you an opportunity to focus on your form and technique. For example, with a bicep curl, a tempo rep would see you raising the dumbbell quickly, then lowering it slowly. This increases the time the muscle is under tension and encourages more muscle growth.

What is zonal training?

The zones referred to are the different zones of the body. My zonal HIIT and strength training work the body in zones – with different muscle areas targeted on different days. This allows you to work a particular muscle group during a 20-minute workout and discover areas of strength and weakness, then rest that group until its turn comes around again, to prevent fatigue and overtraining. It's hard to work out when you are aching, so it is important not to overwork yourself by hammering away at the same areas. Zonal training is a sensible and sustainable way to train if you are training regularly.

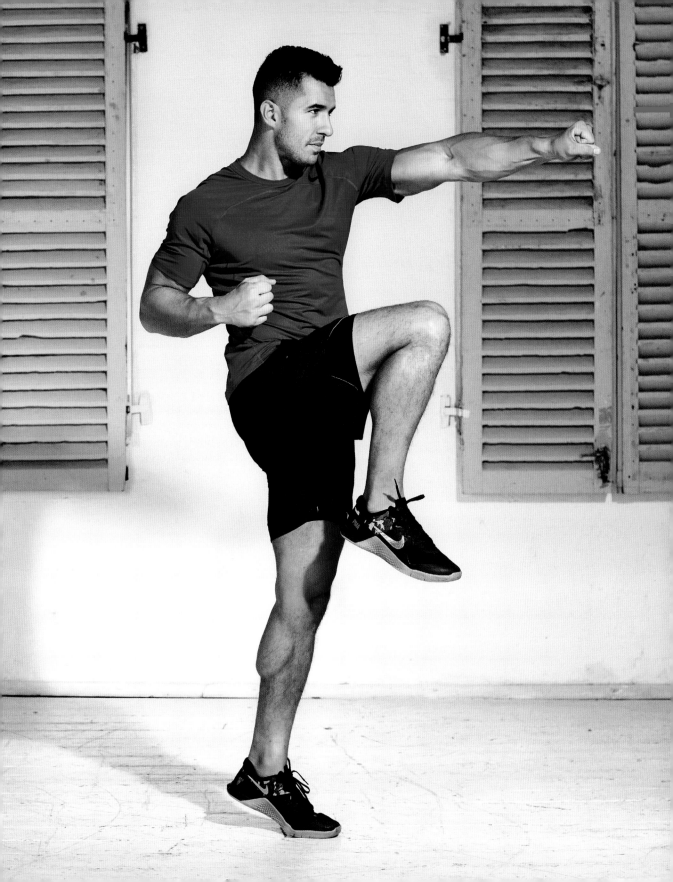

MY TRAINING TIPS

Once you have a training routine in place, you are well on your way, but getting there in the first place can be tricky if you have no idea where to start. The following tips will help you prepare for the challenge of establishing a regular training routine.

IDENTIFY YOUR GOALS

What do you want to achieve with your training and why? Post your goals up somewhere in the house where you can see them, or use them as a screensaver to keep yourself on track.

GYM PREP

It's good to start every workout with a plan, know how long you're training for, what areas you're working and what you want to achieve, so you stay focused on the job in hand. (This is built into the two-week workout plan – *see* chapter 4).

SCHEDULE YOUR TRAINING

Put your workouts and rest day in the diary just like you would meetings and social events and stick to them. If your training isn't in the diary ahead of time you may be reluctant to prioritize it. Scheduling workouts will also help you plan your post-workout meals more effectively.

MAKE SMALL CHANGES

Get active in every area of your life with small changes. Always take the stairs or walk up every escalator, squat while the kettle boils, and get up and sit back down during the ad break of your favourite TV show.

TRACK YOUR PROGRESS

Tracking your progress is not about measuring your weight or waistline. This is about the important things – how fit and healthy you are, and how you feel from the inside out. The other stuff naturally follows if you focus on your food, fitness and PMA journey primarily. Use a training diary (*see* pages 38–9) to track your progress. Whenever you feel disheartened, looking back on this diary will show you exactly how far you've come.

BE PATIENT

Be realistic about the time it takes to see improvement. You need a good 12 weeks of honest training and eating to see real results, so trust the process. Remember, just because you can't immediately see the changes, it does not mean they're not happening.

LOSE THE GYMTIMIDATION

We were all beginners once, so don't worry and believe me when I say nobody is judging you. If you use a gym, use my workouts as a training plan while you are there to give you confidence in the fact you're doing the right thing. If it feels too intimidating, do my routines at home and that confidence will soon be sky high.

DON'T FEAR YOUR WEAKNESSES

If you are not good at something, that's reason enough to keep doing it. Get to know your weaknesses and work to make them your strengths.

FASTED TRAINING

If you are like a certain person I live with and an absolute monster in the mornings, then fasted training isn't for you, but I love to schedule my training first thing in the morning before I've eaten. There are many schools of thought on this but the theory behind it, in very simple terms, is that when your body is in a fasted state, it turns to those stubborn fat stores for energy. Aside from all the possible fat-burning benefits, getting my workout in early sets me up for the day in a positive mindset and it means I can enjoy some nice carbs for my breakfast after I've trained.

I would say that whether you train fasted or not comes down to personal choice and how you perform personally, so again, listen to your body and do what is right for you. I can only tell you what works for me.

HYDRATION

Water is your friend. Everything in your body works better if you are hydrated. It boosts metabolism, aids muscle repair, improves digestion and helps circulation. It also helps when you're trying to lose weight because it helps you to feel full.

Everyone is different in terms of how much water they need to drink each day. Here is a little formula that may help you:

YOUR BODY WEIGHT IN KILOGRAMS DIVIDED BY 30 = YOUR SUGGESTED DAILY WATER INTAKE IN LITRES.

ADD ANOTHER 350ML (12FL OZ) TO YOUR QUOTA FOR EVERY 30 MINUTES THAT YOU WORK OUT.

LAY OUT YOUR WORKOUT GEAR THE NIGHT BEFORE

If, like me, you plan to work out first thing in the mornings, have your clothes prepared and place your alarm across the room so you have to get out of bed to turn it off.

BIN THE SCALES

Measuring your weight is misleading and can hinder progress. Focus on how you look and feel instead. Your weight can go up as you gain muscle, even when your body fat reduces, so step away from those scales! Weekly photographs will give a more honest reflection of your journey, so get snapping.

INVEST IN SOME DUMBBELLS

Get training gear you feel comfortable in and buy a set of dumbbells so you can complete my workouts. Remember to look at your health as an investment, rather than an expense – health is wealth! Dumbbells are available to buy online inexpensively these days. I recommend hexagon-ended dumbbells if possible as they give more stability during floor exercises and won't roll around, but others work fine too. In terms of weights, I advise beginners to use 2.5–4kg (5½–9lb), intermediates to use 4–7.5kg (9–16½lb), and advanced to use 7.5–12.5kg (16½–27½lb).

RECRUIT YOUR FRIENDS

Everything is easier with support. Start an email chain or texting group with your friends or plan a weekly walk to update each other on your progress, share recipes or train together. Having a "fitfam" around you is a great dose of extra motivation.

STRETCH AND RECOVER

Stay on top of your cool downs (*see* pages 122-7) to prevent injury and get the most out of your training plan. It may not be as much fun as jumping around to music and pumping weights, but it is absolutely vital to your progress. You should stretch after every single session.

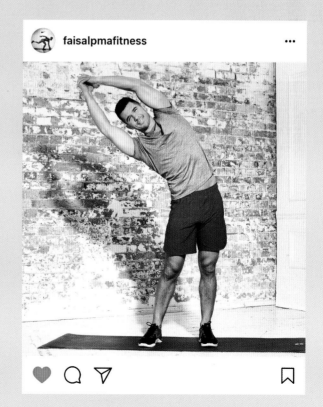

faisalpmafitness

YOUR TRAINING SCHEDULE

Establishing and maintaining a training regime won't be a breeze, but that is what separates those who really want it from those who don't. There is no magic wand here – be prepared to work hard, but that doesn't mean you can't have fun along the way. Before you know it, working out will shift from something you have to do to something you want to do.

If you are serious about getting results, you should try to complete six training sessions a week. That may sound like a lot, but each session is only 20 minutes long and, with 1440 minutes in a day, that's only 1.75 per cent of your entire day. With that in mind, if you are STILL finding excuses like "I don't have time", you need to work on your PMA (*see* chapter 1)!

The more muscle you build, the more calories your body will naturally burn on its own each day so you will find, as you approach or reach your target, that you can reduce your training sessions (if you want to) to just four or five a week.

If you are worried about doing too much when starting out, then try four days a week and work up to the six-day cycle. In this case, follow days one, two, four and five of the weekly training schedule (*see* opposite).

40/20

All of my workouts last for 20 minutes and are made up of 20 exercises, each lasting 40 seconds, followed by 20 seconds of rest. Now, that isn't scary, is it? In fact, the 40/20 formula is an important part of my training.

The beauty of my workouts is that you work to your own personal ability, whether you're a beginner or more advanced. It doesn't matter if you aren't super fit to begin with, just give each exercise everything you've got for those 40 seconds. Slow it right down if you need to; just keep going. If a move is too hard, check if there is a modified version provided for beginners. If it is still too hard, jog or bounce on the spot, or try it with 30 seconds on and 30 seconds off instead. Just keep moving! You may be able to do only five squats in 40 seconds, but this will increase as your fitness levels improve, so track your progress over time.

Weekly plan

I start my training cycle on a Monday, but you can choose whatever day works best for you. What is non-negotiable is your rest day. You must take one full rest day a week to allow your body to recover. Overtraining and under-recovering are two of the biggest mistakes you can make on a fitness journey. Training too much can cause you to plateau, while not resting enough can cause you to burn out. We are in this for the long game, so whether you like it or not, rest is part of the programme.

If you train my way using the two-week workout plan in chapter 4, you will be exercising a different part of your body each day of the week, as outlined opposite.

Day seven / Sunday

Reeeecover! Sunday is a day of rest so don't try to get clever by squeezing in an extra workout on this day. You need that rest for good reason. It will help to prevent injuries and encourage your body to rebuild and recover. Use day seven to sleep, relax and do whatever it is that makes you happy. Sunday is also the perfect day for a cheat day and this is when I like to dive into the chocolates. Make Sunday your fun day every week and it will motivate you to keep on your journey. Remember, when you have your rest and cheat day is flexible, so fit it into a day that best suits your schedule.

Two-week plan

There are detailed and illustrated instructions showing how to perform my workouts in chapter 4. I've outlined which workout to do on each day of weeks one and two. You can either follow the instructions contained in the book for each workout or join me online each day by scanning the first image of each workout with your smartphone to be taken to timed videos of the workouts (*see* instructions, opposite).

SEE IT, SHAZAM IT!

For online access to the workouts in this book, follow these instructions:

1. Download the Android and Apple Shazam app from Shazam.com or the App store.
2. Open the Shazam app.
3. Tap the camera icon in Shazam.
4. In each workout, look for the image with the Shazam logo at the start of the workout.
5. Point your phone's camera at the image with the full image in focus.
6. You will instantly unlock online versions of the workouts in this book.

OPEN **SHAZAM**   TAP **CAMERA**   **SCAN** CODE

"Faisal is genuinely this positive, kind and generous. He is encouraging. He makes you feel like you can do more. He is your greatest ally. He wants you to be your best. Not compared to anyone else. It's hard to fully put into words the impact he has had on my life but it has been measurable and profound. He takes the power of positivity to another level and is absolutely leading by example every single day. He showed me what is possible. And it is nothing to do with who you are or where you come from. It is realistic and attainable. In what often feels like a relentlessly negative world, full of bad news and conflict, Faisal's contagious and empowering positivity is something that I am thankful for every single day."

Gina LoBuglio, 49, San Francisco Supermum

YOUR WEEKLY TRAINING SCHEDULE

DAY ONE / MONDAY:
ARMS AND ABS

DAY TWO / TUESDAY:
LEGS AND BUTT

DAY THREE / WEDNESDAY:
CHEST, BACK AND CORE

DAY FOUR / THURSDAY:
ABS AND CORE

DAY FIVE / FRIDAY:
FULL BODY WITH WEIGHTS

DAY SIX / SATURDAY:
FULL BODY, NO WEIGHTS

DAY SEVEN / SUNDAY:
REST DAY

MYTHS AND MISTAKES DEBUNKED

"Lifting weights will make me bulky."

Stronger doesn't always mean bigger, particularly for women, who don't have the testosterone levels to bulk up like men do. These workouts are designed to make you strong, toned and lean, not to turn you into Arnold Schwarzenegger. You need to lift heavy to build that kind of muscle. Maintaining lean muscle mass requires more energy so you will burn more calories at rest – bulky is not the aim of this programme.

"I only want to lose the fat on the back of my arms."

Unfortunately, you cannot spot-reduce fat and choose the areas to target. We all have different body shapes, which store weight in different areas, and we lose it from different places in different orders. You need to focus on the whole package and trust that you will eventually lose it from where you want. Eating well and performing strength exercises targeting problem areas will help you gain the results you want.

"I need to do cardio for an hour to lose weight."

Wrong. Exercise has moved on from the days where people would try to lose weight by jogging on a treadmill for two hours. The rising popularity of HIIT and strength training shows busy people how effective training for just a short length of time can be.

"I can't afford a gym membership so I will never get in shape."

You don't need a gym to work out. My workouts can be completed almost anywhere. If you are tight for space at home, take your workout to your local park. The world is your gym.

"I'm too old for strength training."

Age is just a number. Strength training can improve bone density, balance, heart health and mobility. The NHS actually recommends over-65s should strength train the major muscle groups two or more times a week. The more you do it, the more you will feel its benefits.

"I need to exercise every day if I want to get quick results."

Overtraining and under-recovering is counterproductive and can do more harm than good. Working out involves your muscle fibres being broken down and then rebuilt, but for that process to take place effectively, you need time to recover. Take that rest day once a week.

"I've put on weight – I'm getting fatter."

Not necessarily, which is why I told you to throw out the bathroom scales! Initially, your increase in muscle mass can outpace your fat loss, so relax. Instagram is full of body transformation photos showing people who look incredible but have actually gained weight in terms of numbers on the scales, because they have added so much muscle definition.

BEFORE YOU BEGIN

Before you start your first day's training, take the Four-move Challenge below to give yourself a little fitness test, and record your results in your training diary (*see pages 38–9*). After that, take the test again each Challenge Wednesday and fill out your results in the "progress report" column. Feel free to take this challenge any day of the week when you want to check your progress or fancy tagging a little extra on at the end of your workout.

THE FOUR–MOVE CHALLENGE

Each exercise covers a key area of strength or endurance. You should always be focused on these areas rather than the numbers on the scales, because these are the improvements you should be striving for.

Wall squat hold: ____ seconds
The challenge: Lean against a wall and squat with your knees at a 90-degree angle, as if you are sitting on a chair. Keep your back against the wall and your arms out in front of you. At no time should your hands touch your knees or the wall. Time how long you can hold the position for.

Plank hold: ____ seconds
The challenge: Hold an elbow plank or a high plank (see page 72) for as long as you can. How long can you hold the position without dropping to the floor or dropping your lower back and losing the plank position?

Push-ups in 30 seconds: ____ push-ups
The challenge: How many push-ups (see page 94) can you do within 30 seconds, on your feet or on your knees? You must kiss the floor with your chest on every rep.

Burpees in 30 seconds: ____ burpees
The challenge: How many burpees (see page 115) can you do within 30 seconds, choosing the beginner or advanced variation?

Well done! That is the very first part of your training journey completed. Don't feel disheartened if you did not do as well as you had hoped because the whole point of this journey is to grow and improve. If you did better than you expected then that right there is lesson number one – never underestimate yourself!

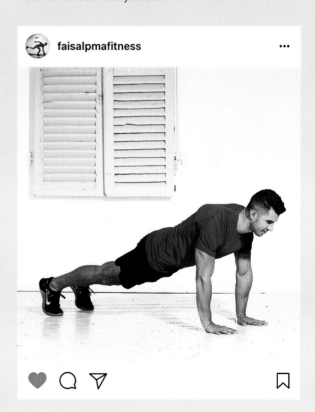

faisalpmafitness

THE TRAINING DIARY

A training diary will help you track your progress – it's helpful and motivating to see how far you've come. Use it to record which days you have trained, which workout you did, any personal bests, anything you did well and areas you think need improving. Your training diary needs to work for you, so play around with it, using the example opposite as a starting point, until you find the best way to record your progress.

You can also use the diary to focus on your daily positive affirmations (*see* page 20) and your weekly goals (for example, doing a training session without stopping or dropping your mid-morning snack), which you will set each Friday and monitor throughout the week. By monitoring your goals daily, you can focus on them closely and build a plan to achieve them if you are veering off course. These goals can be about fitness and exercise, but they should also cover your general wellness – how much sleep you are getting, how much water you are drinking, how positively you are thinking.

Once a week, on Challenge Wednesday, complete a Four-move Challenge (*see* page 37) on top of your normal workout. Note down your results in your training diary so you can see your week-by-week progress at a glance.

YOUR TRAINING COMPANION

I know that the hardest part is the start, when you're learning to integrate training into your life, so on the following pages, I will talk you through each day of your first two weeks of training (*see* pages 40–3) and you can train alongside me online for extra motivation. I want to help you to stay motivated on the programme, but also to help you get into the habit of focusing on all three sides of the PMA Method pyramid (*see* page 10) – PMA, food and fitness. The aim is for you to reset your thinking, eating and training habits during this time.

Now you are ready to start day one. Forget all your past mistakes; this is a clean slate, a fresh start, and day one on the journey to becoming the absolute best version of yourself. Don't forget to use your training diary to stay on track. Turn to your first workout (*see* pages 46–57), smash it out and then grab a pen to fill out day one of your diary. Wishing you love, luck, success and PMA, guys. Go and get it!

	WORKOUT COMPLETED	WORKOUT EVALUATION
DAY ONE/ MONDAY	eg) 20-minute arms and abs in the gym	eg) Felt strong on the bicep curls but stopped twice during the burpees
DAY TWO/ TUESDAY		
DAY THREE/ WEDNESDAY		
DAY FOUR/ THURSDAY		
DAY FIVE/ FRIDAY		
DAY SIX/ SATURDAY		

OTHER EXERCISE	GOAL-TRACKING	FOOD	PROGRESS REPORT
eg) Walked up all the escalators on the tube on the way to work and walked home instead of getting the bus	eg) Hit my goal of sleeping for 8 hours. Did not drink my 2 litres of water. Will bring a big bottle to work tomorrow	eg) Ate well for lunch and dinner but ate carbs for breakfast without working out and succumbed to a chocolate bar at 3pm	eg) Personal bests, achievements and Four-move Challenge results

WEEK ONE

	DAY ONE/MONDAY MOTIVATION MONDAY	**DAY TWO/TUESDAY** TARGET TUESDAY	**DAY THREE/WEDNESDAY** CHALLENGE WEDNESDAY
YOUR PMA	Start as you mean to go on because your mood on a Monday morning can set your mood for the whole week. As soon as you wake up, think of at least one reason why you feel great and repeat that positive affirmation out loud to yourself at least five times. Say that affirmation to yourself throughout the day when negativity tries to creep in.	Day one is out of the way – well done! To keep you going, ask yourself what is my why (see page 18)? Think of three whys – why do you want to eat healthier, train harder and think more positively? – and write them down. Stick your whys somewhere you can see them or save them as the background on your phone and read them throughout the day. They may change as you get fitter and your mindset shifts, so revisit them each Tuesday and write new ones when they change.	You're half way there! It's Challenge Wednesday so it's time to take your weekly Wednesday challenge (see page 37). There is nothing more motivating than a PB, so go get it! If your PMA levels are slipping with the dreaded hump-day blues, turn back to pages 14–21 and have a flick through the PMA chapter again. We all need a little recharge now and again, so give it a quick read and then give yourself a little pep talk!
YOUR WORKOUT	Set your alarm half an hour early and smash out my 20-minute high-energy arms and abs workout (see pages 46–57). An awesome workout first thing on a Monday ensures your week begins on a high. Save your breakfast until afterwards and do this workout fasted for maximum impact.	Move over Kim Kardashian, we've got this! It's time to hit those legs and butts with a 20-minute lower body session (see pages 58–69). You will find that the stronger your legs get, the easier other exercises become and that, ladies and gents, is why we never skip leg day.	Today's 20-minute sweat fest is all about the chest, back and core (see pages 70–83). For you guys, the benefits of chest and back training are more obvious, but for ladies the results aren't as visible. However, honing the muscles in this area will help to streamline the appearance of your upper body and provide you with functional strength, which will help you with everyday movements. It will also help to improve posture which, in turn, helps fight common problems like back pain. So, we are doing it, no arguments!
YOUR FUEL	Fuel your body post-workout with a hearty #MeatfreeMonday breakfast full of protein and that all-essential carb element. How about my Mexican Huevos Rancheros (see page 145)? Make some extra tomato sauce while you're in the kitchen to save cooking time tomorrow. Dish it up on a wholemeal tortilla with half a mashed-up avocado and a squeeze of lime juice. Any leftovers can be eaten for lunch – just lose the tortilla if you haven't smashed out some pre-lunch training.	Try doing your workout fasted again this morning and use up yesterday's extra sauce for another portion of Mexican Huevos Rancheros.	Your muscles will be feeling tired by now so make sure you're getting in lots of protein and amino acids to speed up that muscle repair and recovery. The frittatas are calling. Try one of my frittata recipes (see pages 142–4) for breakfast or lunch today, but don't forget to make extra to see you through breakfast and lunch tomorrow.

DAY FOUR/THURSDAY
TRANSFORMATION THURSDAY

Let's call this Transformation Thursday, because who doesn't love a bit of alliteration? It takes a while to see changes in your body. That is normal, so don't get frustrated and give up. Get into the habit of taking a photo in the same pose on your phone after each Thursday workout. Soon enough you will see the changes, which will spur you on to keep going.

Are you ready to get hardCORE? Turn to pages 84–91 for some sweaty interval and strength sets to get that core burning. We all love a toned tummy, but the benefits of a strong core extend much deeper. Your core is your body's powerhouse. Strengthening it can help prevent injuries and back pain, and improve balance and stability.

Treat yourself to my Fire-on-fire Chicken Madras tonight (see page 194). Just throw everything into a pan and let it roast away while you enjoy a relaxing evening. Take a salt bath or stretch out those muscles while your dinner cooks so your body is primed for your final two days of training. For a great alternative veggie one-pot dish, try Mrs PMA's Cauliflower and Paneer Coconut Curry (see page 182).

DAY FIVE/FRIDAY
GOAL-SETTING FRIDAY

Take 10 minutes for yourself every Friday somewhere quiet to reconnect with your journey. Use your training diary to assess this week's achievements. What was hard? How did you overcome it? Which exercises did you perform well? Which areas need improving? Were there any days on which you ate something you wished you hadn't? Now identify three goals you would like to achieve next week, so that you start again after the weekend with clear focus.

Today's full-body session with weights (see pages 92–107) is about the full package. Being healthy is about being strong. A strong body creates a strong mind and vice versa. And muscles burn more calories than fat, so don't skip your strength sessions if you're serious about results. Look yourself in the mirror and psyche yourself up for this. Trust me, it works! Tell yourself you are going to give it every last drop and really go for it. I want you to go hell for leather like never before.

It is the end of the week and you're thrilled it's over! So, after work, dinner or drinks sound tempting. Don't deprive yourself, it's okay to go out, just make good choices when you're there. Try to schedule your training later in the day (before dinner) so you can order carbs with your meal when you are out and relax a bit. However, do your very best to avoid alcohol – those empty calories are undoing your efforts. Is it really worth it after all the hard work you have put in this week?

DAY SIX/SATURDAY
SOCIAL SATURDAY

The weekend is here! Holding Social Saturdays will inject some extra PMA into your life. Start a group message with your fit friends or buddies who are on the same journey as you, or arrange a weekly walk to update each other. Sharing progress reports each Saturday will help to motivate each other, as you are accountable to someone other than yourself. It is so much easier to stick to a plan when you have support from friends and, sometimes, the added competition drives you on.

Turn to pages 108–15 for today's full-body session without weights, which is a boxing-inspired workout to help you punch away the aggression and stresses of the week and start the weekend feeling invincible. Don't worry if you have never boxed before – these are simple drills to get you moving quickly and explosively. This is a fun workout to do with friends on a Social Saturday, and it's equipment free, so you can do it anywhere.

It's Saturday night and the chances are you are craving a big old Thai takeaway. Eating out can be hard when you're trying to be good so why not eat at home and invite your friends over for a Saturday night Fakeaway? Perhaps you and your pals could take it in turns hosting a weekly supper club with your favourite #FaisalFakeaway recipes, to avoid the temptations of eating out? Mrs PMA's Thai Turkey Burgers with Almond Butter Satay Sauce are always a winner (see page 176).

WEEK TWO

	DAY ONE/MONDAY MOTIVATION MONDAY	**DAY TWO/TUESDAY** TARGET TUESDAY	**DAY THREE/WEDNESDAY** CHALLENGE WEDNESDAY
YOUR PMA	Firstly, don't forget to continue with your positive affirmations every morning. It is important that you don't let them slide. Now, turn back to the goals you wrote down in your training diary on Friday. Focus on working towards them this week. Whether it is doing a training session without stopping, sleeping eight hours a night or dropping your mid-morning snack, think carefully about the steps you are going to take this week to make sure you achieve them.	Now you are in week two, think about your reserve tank. We can always push harder than we think and our mind gives up before our body, so think about how much you want to place in your reserve tank before you start out. If you feel like giving up on an exercise today, remember how many extra reps you placed in the tank. When you go to stop because you feel exhausted, squeeze out the extra reps you promised yourself. Don't give up until you have emptied that tank!	If you hit the mid-week slump today, negative thoughts may creep in. If you have a bad day or things are getting you down, take some time at the end of the day to take a pen and paper, or take out your phone, and write down all the positives about your day. What did you learn? How can you use this knowledge in the future? The worst thing you can do is ignore things and let them build up internally, so this is a useful exercise to help you to dust down your thoughts – like spring-cleaning your mind.
YOUR WORKOUT	We are back on those arms and abs today (*see* page 116). Lay out your gym gear the night before so you can get this one done early before breakfast. Arm workouts are the perfect opportunity to perfect those tempo reps with your dumbbells, so let's focus on slowing down those movements and combining explosive movements with slower ones, to get right into those muscle fibres.	We are back to those legs and butts today so get your legs throbbing and that booty popping. Turn to page 117 for today's 20-minute lower-body blast. Really focus on squeezing those bum cheeks together during your squats today. Try the same with your lunges. Squeezing your butt together helps you lift your body using force from your legs, removing the strain from your lower back. It also encourages you to lock out fully at the top of the movement.	It is time to put your back into it – literally. Turn to page 118 for today's chest, back and core extravaganza. Today is also Challenge Wednesday (*see* page 37), so update your challenge record in your training diary and see if you have improved in any areas. It is still very early days, and this is just the start of your journey, so do not expect miracles. Just keep recording your progress every Wednesday and trust the process.
YOUR FUEL	A decent post-workout breakfast will refuel you nicely and set you up until lunch. Try my Turmeric Scrambled Eggs with Roasted Tomatoes (*see* page 135), serving it on a slice of toasted rye bread to get in that magical combo of carbs and protein. If you had a cheat day on Sunday, why not try a little detox today and do your small part for the planet with a #MeatfreeMonday?	Training your legs requires lots of energy so you may find yourself more peckish than normal today. Get in a good dose of protein and carbs post-workout, such as my Baba's Beef Kofte in a wholemeal pitta (*see* page 156). Prepare some healthy snacks as well, so you don't cave in mid-afternoon if the hunger strikes. A boiled egg or spicy nuts are a great snack and full of good fats. If you are craving something sweeter, a handful of raspberries or strawberries should do the trick.	Why not try my tasty Courgetti Bologneasy for dinner tonight (*see* page 193)? If you are eating it post-workout you can replace the courgetti with some wholemeal spaghetti for a good dose of carbs. Alternatively, have a go at my super-simple Garlic Flatbreads. Try them once and you'll never look back!

DAY FOUR/THURSDAY
TRANSFORMATION THURSDAY

Remember to take your Thursday photo to track your progress. You may not want to share this because it's an intimate thing, but why not share other parts of your journey? The online community can be incredibly supportive; you feel part of a family because you are all in it together. Sharing your food choices and training publicly and honestly may also help keep you on track because you know people are watching. If you use the hashtag #PMAMethod I will be able to follow your journey, too.

Are you ready for another 20 minutes of core and abs? The waistline is a problem area for a lot of people and while you can't pick and choose where you lose fat from, you can work on toning the area to improve its appearance. The HIIT and strength element of the workout on page 119 is great for overall fat burning too, so let's go hard or go home!

Try your workout in the evening if you can, and marinate some miso salmon (see page 175) as you train, then add the carb option with some brown rice. Double your portions to adhere to the cook once, eat twice ethos. Refrigerate the extras and enjoy them for a ready-made lunch tomorrow.

DAY FIVE/FRIDAY
GOAL-SETTING FRIDAY

It is time to set those goals again. Think about how your week has gone and what has and hasn't gone well. Note down your thoughts in your training diary. Reflect on the three goals you set last Friday. Have you smashed them? If so, well done! Feels amazing, right? Now think of three new goals for the following week. If you haven't reached your goals yet, hopefully, in working towards them you are one step closer, so think carefully about how you will get even closer in this following week.

Are you ready to get your strong on? Today's full-body session with weights (see page 120) will hit those muscles! Nothing looks as good as strong feels, so really embrace these sessions. Strong is the new sexy, so pick up those dumbbells and give this workout everything you've got. I always find weighted sessions more effective in front of a mirror, so give it a go if you can. There's a lot to be said for looking yourself in the eye and daring yourself not to give up during a workout.

Try to smash out another fasted session this morning so you can go big at breakfast. A decent brekkie at the end of the week always feels great. How about a big old chocolate protein pancake stack (see page 132)? If the thought of that doesn't get you through a workout, nothing will! Lunch today should be super simple if you're using yesterday's leftovers. Just add that salmon to a nice plate of mixed salad.

DAY SIX/SATURDAY
SOCIAL SATURDAY

The weekend is here! Just one session left before you rest and recover. Let's try something different this Social Saturday. Grab your friends, family or partner and go for an outdoor run before today's session. If you don't regularly run outdoors it can be strangely daunting, but it's time to get comfortable with being uncomfortable because life begins at the end of your comfort zone! Record your run distance and time in your training diary so you can see how it improves as you continue.

As it's Social Saturday, why not do today's full-body session without weights (see page 121) in the gym or your local park with your friends? Or invite them round to smash it out with you at home? Fitness should be fun and we are stronger together. I love working out in a group as it brings out the best in me. Saturday's sessions are always equipment free so you can take them anywhere and get social. Go for a nice long walk before or after your session as part of your warm up or cool down and make a day of it.

Get your friends or family together again for supper club week two and cook up another Saturday night Fakeaway. My version of Chicken Katsu Curry with Egg-fried Cauliflower Rice is an absolute winner if you're looking for some dinspiration (see pages 188–9).

CHAPTER 4

TWO-WEEK WORKOUT PLAN

Here's your drill. Your training schedule is one 20-minute workout every day for six days in a row, one day off. You'll have a new session each day for two weeks, then you repeat the cycle. And you give it 100 per cent in each short session.

All sessions are done to time rather than reps so that you can work to your own ability. 20 minutes of your absolute best looks the same regardless of how fit you are. If you are a complete beginner and find these exercises too hard, there are beginner options for many of them that you can try until you are ready to progress, or consider a four-day weekly cycle (*see* page 34).

Remember, there are 20 moves in every workout. Each move lasts 40 seconds and then you get 20 seconds of rest before moving on to the next one. If you are struggling with the 40/20 formula, adapt it to 30 seconds of work, 30 seconds of rest, but at least try 40/20 before you decide it's too difficult. It is supposed to be hard and you are supposed to feel tired and challenged – that's the whole point! Use a clock or your phone to time your workouts. There are specialist timer apps that you can download, which will bleep when your 40 seconds is up and again when your next exercise is due to begin. This allows you to focus entirely on your workout without worrying about the time.

Dynamic warm-ups are written into each workout, and I highly recommend you cool down after every single workout. If you don't stretch adequately, you will feel it the next day, believe me! Complete my recovery sequence on pages 122–7 as a bare minimum. You can also access my workouts online – that way you can train side-by-side with me, which is great for those days when you need a morale boost. Look out for the Shazam codes (*see* page 35), which you can scan with your phone.

Before you start, briefly read through all the exercise descriptions and try a couple of reps on any that are new to you, so you can apply yourself to the 40 second on, 20 second off rule effectively.

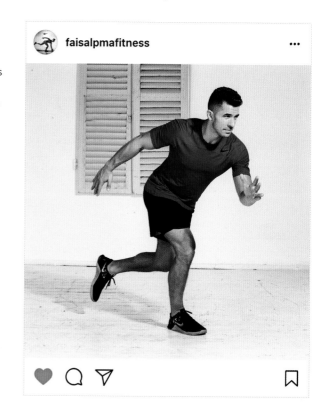

faisalpmafitness

I could have designed workouts you could do anywhere with no equipment, but I felt like I'd be short-changing you if I didn't write the best workout plans possible. Body-weighted HIIT is fantastic, but I was keen to up the ante and provide an extra element and opportunity for development in the form of strength training.

For that reason, almost all of my workouts require a set of dumbbells. If you are following this plan at home rather than the gym, that is the only equipment you will need to buy. You can pick them up cheaply online (*see* page 33).

If you are travelling to somewhere with no gym, a lot of the dumbbell exercises can be done with an easy-to-pack resistant band instead. Alternatively, you can do just the body-weighted exercises and repeat them for the full 20-minute session.

"PMA has been so powerful because it makes us aware of the power of our minds and attitudes. These are things that can never be trained enough and that is the beauty of PMA. It becomes who you are. It's learning to dig deep until we encounter that person inside of us, who is much stronger than we ever knew. It's the ability to take control of any situation, realising it's not what happens to you that matters, it's how you choose to respond. Over time with Faisal, I've realised that if you can tap into your PMA, anything is possible."

Maria Fernanda Rodas, 28, Miami

EQUIPMENT: ONE SET OF DUMBBELLS AND A TIMER

WORKOUT LENGTH: 20 MINUTES

EXERCISES: 20 MOVES

EXERCISE LENGTH: 40 SECONDS ON / 20 SECONDS OFF

DUMBBELL GUIDE:
BEGINNER 2.5–4KG (5½–9LB)
INTERMEDIATE: 4–7.5KG (9–16½LB)
ADVANCED: 7.5–12.5KG (16½–27½LB)

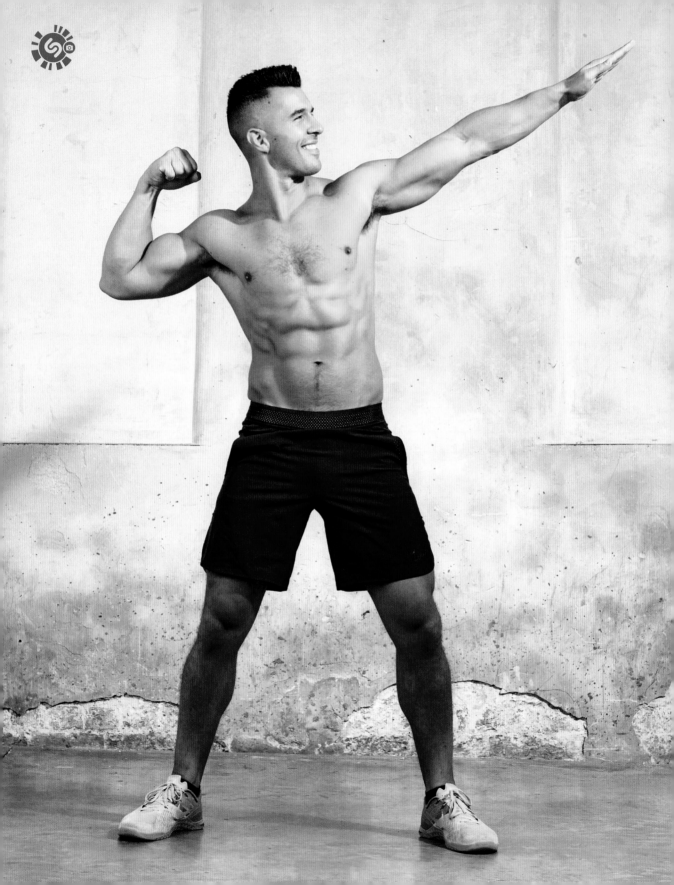

WEEK ONE
DAY ONE/MONDAY
ARMS AND ABS

1. WALKOUTS

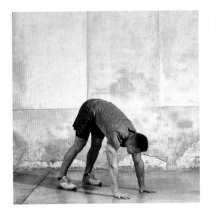 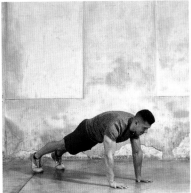

Begin in a standing position. Bend forward at the hips, keeping your legs as straight as possible, and rest your hands on the floor below your shoulders. Now walk your hands out in front of you into push up position. Walk your hands back beneath your shoulders, then uncurl your back one vertebra at a time as you come back up to standing. Repeat.

2. PLANK SHOULDER TAPS

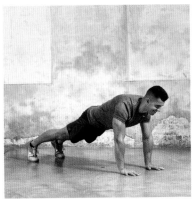 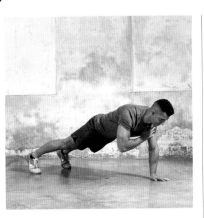 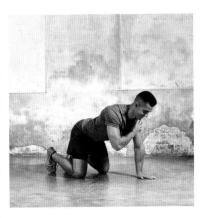

Get into plank position. Tap the left shoulder with the right hand, then return to plank position. Repeat, alternating sides.

TRAINER'S TIP: Keep your hips parallel to the floor and stop them dipping down. Keep your body as stiff as a plank and your core tight and engaged.

BEGINNERS: Drop to your knees if you are struggling with a full plank.

3. PLANK SWIVELS

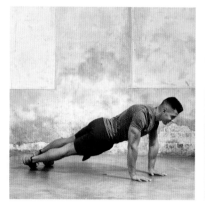 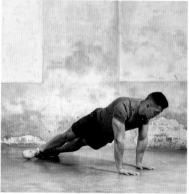 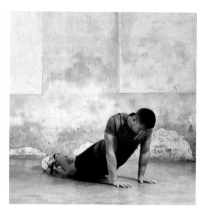

Get into plank position. Keeping your arms and shoulders in place, swivel your hips round so that your right hip is closest to the floor. Return to neutral, then repeat, alternating sides.

TRAINER'S TIP: Your shoulders should be in line with your wrists. Imagine your body as a plank of wood, with everything in straight and in line, to prevent your hips dipping down.

BEGINNERS: Perform this move from a kneeling position, with knees slid back a little.

4. PLANK T-ROTATIONS

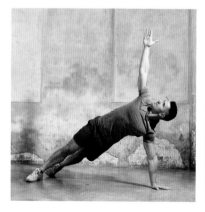 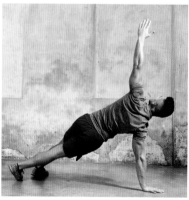 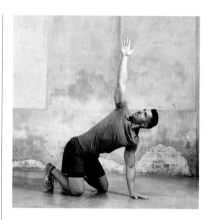

Get into plank position. Rotate your torso toward the right and raise your right hand up toward the ceiling. Return to plank position. Repeat, alternating sides.

TRAINER'S TIP: Follow your hands with your eyes so you look in the direction you are reaching.

BEGINNERS: Drop to your knees if a full plank is too challenging.

5. ALTERNATING JACK KNIVES

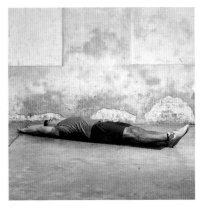 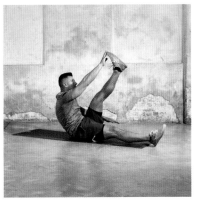 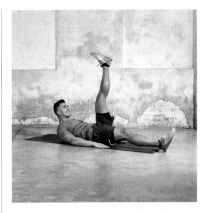

Lie flat on your back with your arms raised above your head. Raise your right leg, and raise your left arm up to meet your right toe, trying to bring your back off the floor. Repeat, alternating sides.

TRAINER'S TIP: Keep your chin on your chest to prevent neck strain. Don't be tempted to use your neck to pull yourself up.

BEGINNERS: Keep your back and arms on the floor while raising your leg.

6. DUMBBELL BICEP CURLS

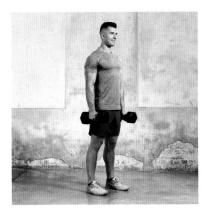 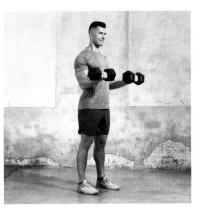 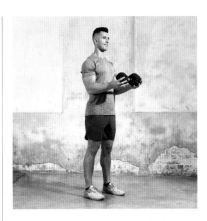

Holding dumbbells, stand with your feet shoulder-width apart and your elbows tucked into your body. Turn your hands so your palms face toward the sky and curl them up toward your shoulders, then back down to your side. Repeat.

TRAINER'S TIP: Make sure you fully extend when curling down, so that your arms are completely straight. Keep your elbows touching the sides of your body throughout the movement, so they don't flare out.

BEGINNERS: Use one weight, holding it at each end in your hands.

7. DUMBBELL KNEELING SHOULDER PRESS

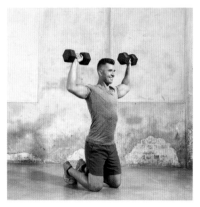 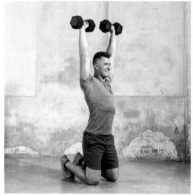 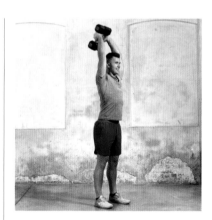

Get into a kneeling position holding dumbbells. Raise your arms outward, with palms facing forward, elbows forming 90° angles. From this starting position, press the weights up, above your head, so that your arms are straight, and then bend your arms back to the starting position. Repeat the movement.

TRAINER'S TIP: Look forward and keep your back straight to prevent arching.

BEGINNERS: Use one weight, holding it at each end in your hands.

8. DUMBBELL OVERHEAD TRICEP EXTENSION

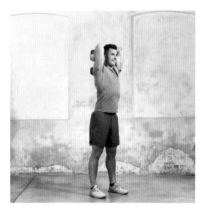 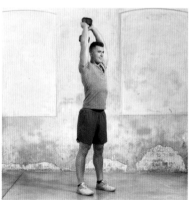

Stand, holding one weight behind your head, with your elbows pointing to the sky beside your head. From this starting position, straighten your elbows to raise the weight above the head, then lower the arms back to the starting position. Repeat.

TRAINER'S TIP: Keep your head looking forward.

ADVANCED: Use two weights and keep them touching throughout the movement.

9. DUMBBELL TRICEP KICK-BACKS

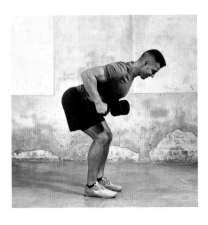

Holding dumbbells, stand in a bent-over position with your feet shoulder-width apart. Keep your back flat, your chest over your toes and your elbows tucked into your sides. Bend your elbows to form a 90° angle. From this starting position, straighten your arms, raising the lower arms backward, then return to the starting position. Repeat.

TRAINER'S TIP: Keep your back flat and stick your bum out behind you.

10. DUMBBELL BICEP CURL TO SHOULDER PRESS

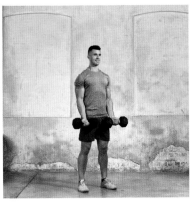

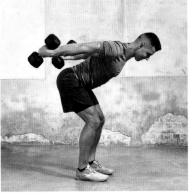

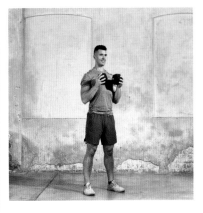

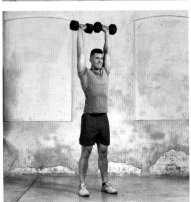

Holding dumbbells, stand with feet shoulder-width apart, elbows tucked into your body and palms facing forward. From this starting position, bicep curl your weights to your shoulders, then twist your wrists so that your palms are facing forwards as you press your weights overhead. Arms and elbows should be locked out above your head. Reverse your movements to bring the dumbbells back to the starting position. Repeat.

BEGINNERS: Use one weight to scale this movement down, holding it at each end.

TRAINER'S TIP: Retain a slight bend in your knees and keep the feet shoulder-width apart.

YOU'RE HALFWAY THERE. KEEP GOING!

11. DUMBBELL RUSSIAN TWISTS

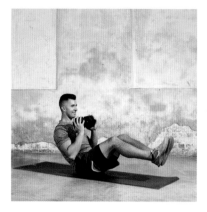 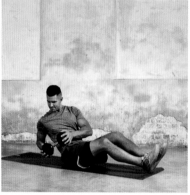 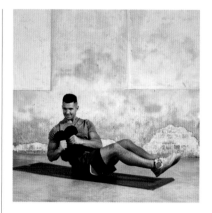

Holding one end of a dumbbell in each hand, sit in a V-sit position with your feet off the floor and knees slightly bent. Rotate the weight from one hip to the other repeatedly.

TRAINER'S TIP: Make sure your chest follows the weight for maximum rotation.

BEGINNERS: Keep your feet on the floor with knees bent.

ADVANCED: Use two weights and keep them touching.

12. DUMBBELL RAISED LEG TOE TOUCHES

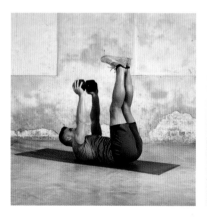 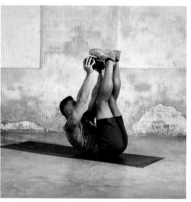 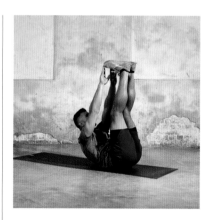

Lie on your back with both legs raised straight up, heels facing the ceiling. Hold one end of a dumbbell in each hand. Roll your shoulders up and off the floor and reach to touch your toes. Return your shoulders to the floor and repeat.

TRAINER'S TIP: Keep your heels facing the ceiling.

BEGINNERS: Try it without the weight.

13. DUMBBELL V-SIT SHOULDER PRESS

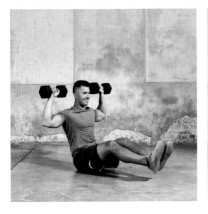 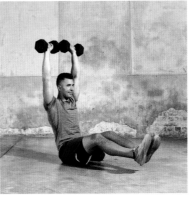 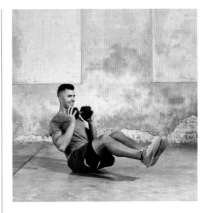

Sit on the floor in a V-sit position, with your feet off the floor and knees slightly bent. Holding a dumbbell in each hand, raise your arms and open them out to the sides, each elbow bent at a 90° angle. From this starting position, straighten the elbows to shoulder press both weights above your head, then lower them back to the starting position and repeat.

TRAINER'S TIP: Keep your palms facing forward.

BEGINNERS: Try the move with one weight. Or hold the V-sit with no weight – start with your hands in front of your chest, then raise them up above your head and return to the starting position.

14. DUMBBELL SIT-UP REACHES

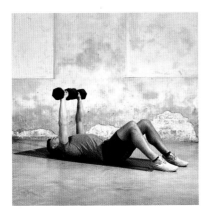 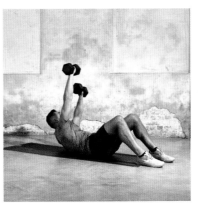 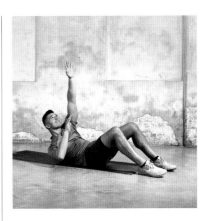

Lie down on the floor with your knees bent and your feet flat on the floor. Hold weights in your hands and extend your arms straight up. Now reach with your right arm straight up toward the ceiling, rotating the torso to the left and rolling the right shoulder blade up off the floor. Repeat, alternating arms, in a continuous movement without resting your shoulders on the floor.

BEGINNERS: Try it without weights.

TRAINER'S TIP: Keep your arms straight and elbows locked out, ensuring you feel the twist in your abs.

15. DUMBBELL PLANK PASSES

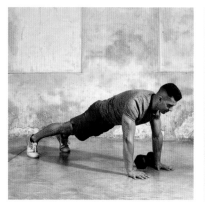 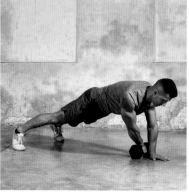 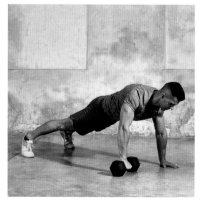

Get into plank position with one weight placed behind your left hand on the floor. Maintaining the plank, raise your right hand off the floor and move it to the left to pick up the weight. Place it beneath your right shoulder, then place your right hand down on the floor in front of the weight. Repeat, alternating sides.

TRAINER'S TIP: Keep your hips parallel to the floor to restrict rotation and don't strain your neck by looking up at a clock. Instead, put a timer on the floor or set a 40-second alarm.

ONLY FIVE MOVES LEFT. LET'S EMPTY THE TANK!

16. DUMBBELL CLOSE GRIP HAMMER CURLS

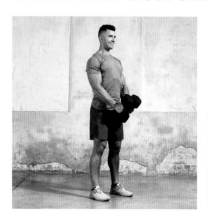 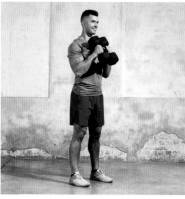

Holding two dumbbells together, stand with your feet shoulder-width apart, your elbows tucked into your body and your palms facing one another, holding each weight like a hammer. From this starting position, keeping your elbows tight to your body, raise your lower arms to curl the weights to your shoulders. Straighten your arms to bring them back down to full extension. Repeat.

TRAINER'S TIP: Press your shoulder blades towards one another and keep your feet shoulder-width apart.

17. DUMBBELL ARNOLD PRESS

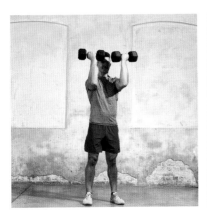 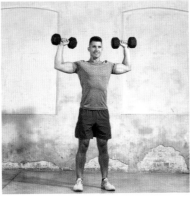 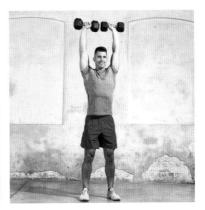

Stand with your feet shoulder-width apart, your elbows raised in front of you at right angles, holding both weights in front of your face with your palms facing you – as though you have your boxing guard up. From this starting position, open out your arms and twist the weights round so that your palms face forward, then straighten your arms to press the weights up. Twist the weights back again as you lower your arms to the starting position.

TRAINER'S TIP: Perform this move slowly and keep your body tight like a plank, with your glutes squeezed.

18. DUMBBELL ALTERNATING TRICEP KICK-BACKS

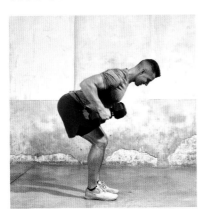 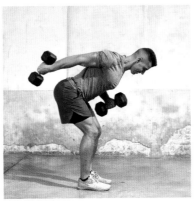 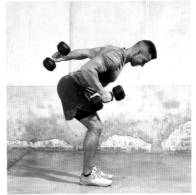

Holding a dumbbell in each hand, stand in a bent-over position with your feet shoulder-width apart. Keep your back flat, your chest over your toes and your elbows tucked into your sides. Bend your elbows to form a 90° angle. From this starting position, straighten your right arm, raising the lower arm backward, then return to the starting position. Repeat, alternating sides.

TRAINER'S TIP: Keep your back flat rather than curved to prevent lower back strain.

19. DUMBBELL PUSH PRESS

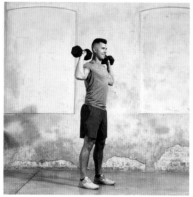

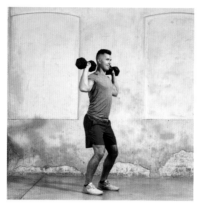

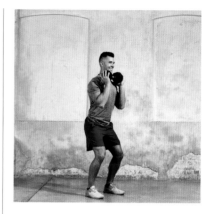

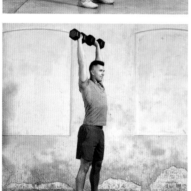

Stand tall, with your feet shoulder-width apart, holding your weights at your shoulders, with your arms open and palms facing forward. In one flowing movement, bend your knees, then lock them out straight, and use the driving force of that straightening motion to press the weights above your head. Bring your arms down to the starting position, then repeat.

BEGINNERS: Use one weight, holding it at each end in your hands.

TRAINER'S TIP: Try to make this a seamless continuous movement.

20. DUMBBELL BICEP CURL TO FOREHEAD

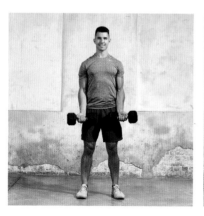

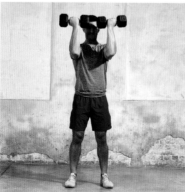

Stand tall, with your feet shoulder-width apart, holding your weights by your sides with your palms facing forward and tucking your elbows into your sides. From this starting position, curl the weights to your forehead, bringing your elbows up away from your body so they follow the weights. Return to the starting position and repeat.

TRAINER'S TIP: Avoid twisting your wrists throughout the movement.

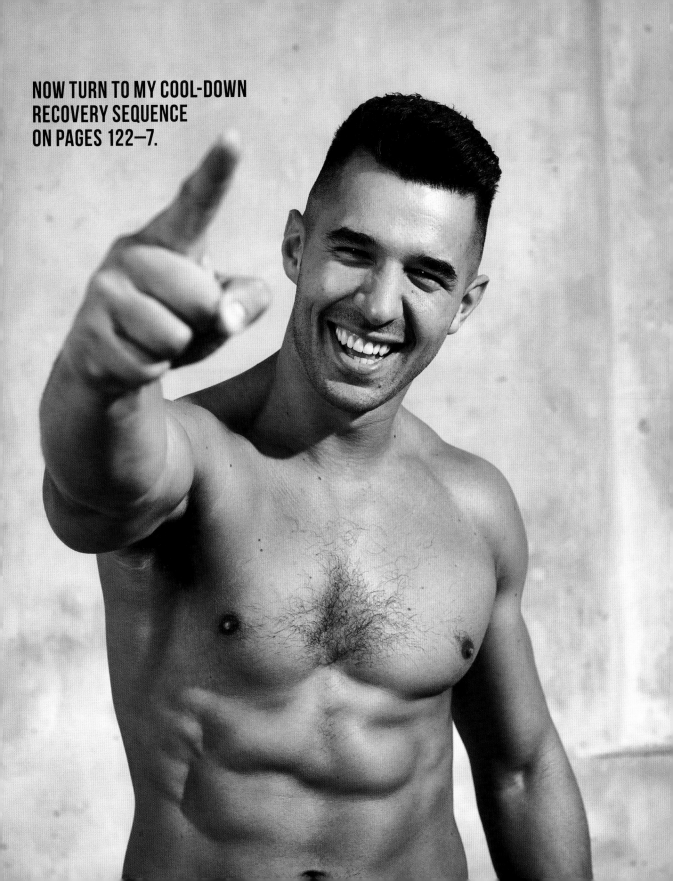

NOW TURN TO MY COOL-DOWN
RECOVERY SEQUENCE
ON PAGES 122–7.

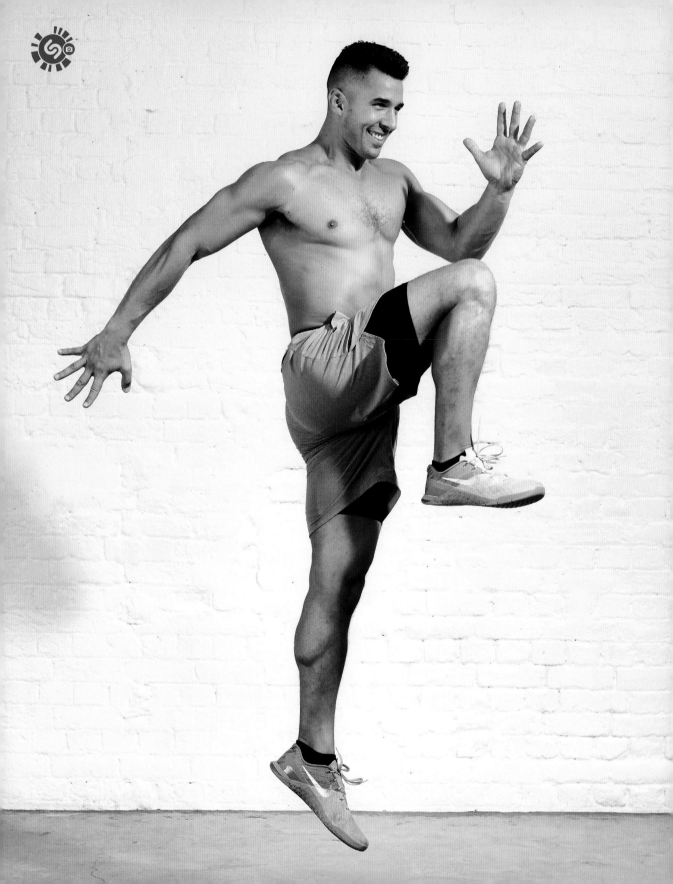

LEGS AND BUTT

1. LUNGES

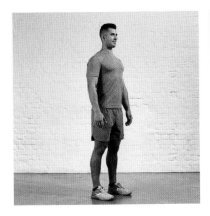 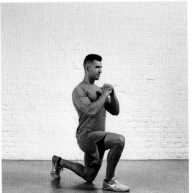

Stand with your feet hip-width apart. Step forward with your right foot and lower your hips to bring your left knee toward the floor, so that both knees are bent at a 90° angle. Drive the weight down through your right heel as you push back up to the starting position. Repeat, alternating legs.

TRAINER'S TIP: Focus on a spot ahead of you when you lunge so you don't lower your head.

2. SQUATS

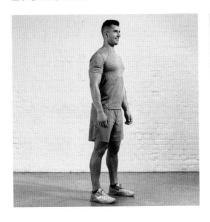 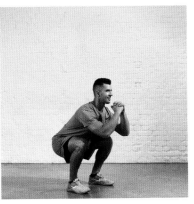

TRAINER'S TIP: Always keep your chest up and back straight, and put all your body weight in your heels. Squeeze your glutes together as you stand as if you are trying to crack an egg with your bum cheeks.

Stand with feet shoulder-width apart. Bend your knees to lower your bum toward your heels, and raise your arms to join your hands in front of your chest. Rise back to standing. Repeat.

3. SIDE LUNGES

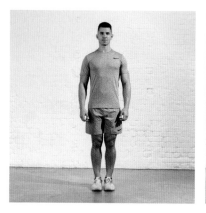 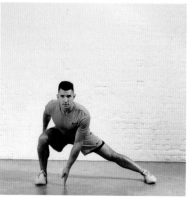

Stand with your feet close together. Step your right leg out to the side and bend your right knee to bring yourself into a squat, keeping your left leg straight. As you lower, bring the fingertips of your left arm to the floor in front of you. Step your right foot back to the left foot and return to standing. Repeat, alternating sides.

TRAINER'S TIP: Keep your standing leg straight when you lunge to the other side, and keep your chest up.

4. TEMPO SQUATS 4-1

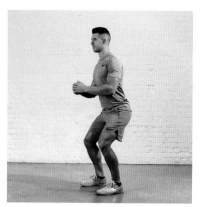 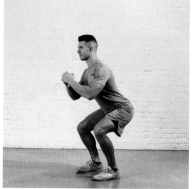

Stand with your feet shoulder-width apart. Perform a standard squat, but this time, lower your body into the squat slowly, to a count of 4 seconds. Rise up explosively to standing to a count of 1 second. Repeat.

TRAINER'S TIP: Keep your chest up and eyes forward. Press your body weight into your heels throughout the movement. Squeeze the glutes as you return to standing.

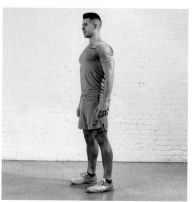

5. CURTSEY LUNGE

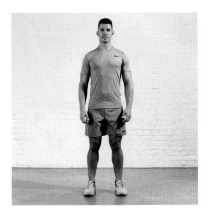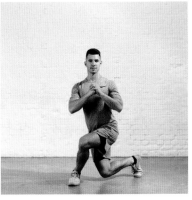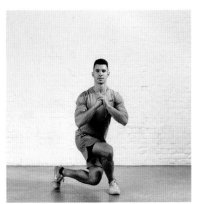

Stand with your feet hip-width apart. Step your right leg toward the left behind your left leg into the lunge, and raise your arms to join your hands in front of your chest. Try to tap your right knee to floor, then return to standing. Repeat, alternating legs.

TRAINER'S TIP: Keep your chest up and imagine you are curtseying to the Queen in front of you.

6. DUMBBELL LUNGES

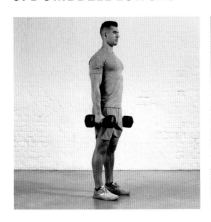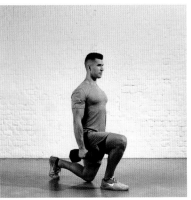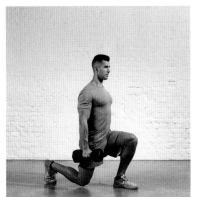

Stand with your feet hip-width apart, holding dumbbells in your hands by your sides. Step your right foot forward and tap your left knee to the floor, then return to standing. Repeat, alternating legs.

TRAINER'S TIP: Always look forward when you lunge and don't step so far out that you lose balance.

7. DUMBBELL SQUATS

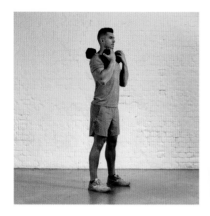 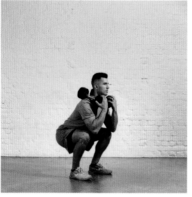 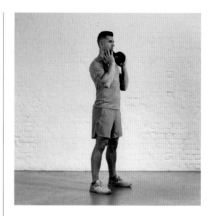

Stand with your feet shoulder-width apart, holding dumbbells on your shoulders as pictured. Bend your knees to lower your body into a squat, bringing your bum toward your heels. Rise back to standing. Repeat.

TRAINER'S TIP: Always keep your chest up and back straight and put all your body weight in your heels.

BEGINNERS: If you are struggling, hold one weight in front of your chest as shown.

8. DUMBBELL SIDE LUNGES

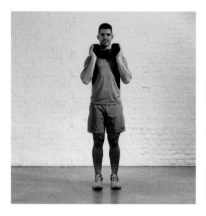 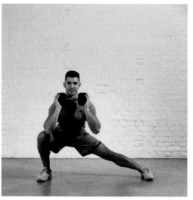 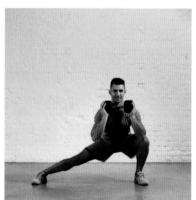

Stand with your feet close together, holding a dumbbell under your chin as shown. Step your right leg out to the side and bend your right knee to bring yourself into a squat, keeping your left leg straight. Step your right foot back to the left foot and bring yourself back to standing. Repeat, alternating sides.

TRAINER'S TIP: Keep the standing leg straight and your chest up as you lunge.

9. DUMBBELL TEMPO SQUATS 4-1

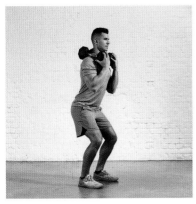

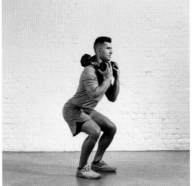

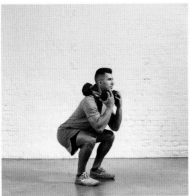

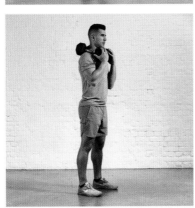

Perform a tempo squat holding a set of dumbbells on your shoulders as shown, to up the ante. Squat down slowly to a count of 4, then push up fast to a count of 1. Repeat.

TRAINER'S TIP: Don't let the dumbbell weights pull your chest forward. Keep the chest high throughout the movement.

10. DUMBBELL CURTSEY LUNGE

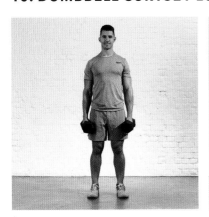

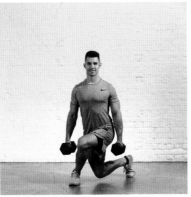

Perform the curtsey lunge holding dumbbells by your sides throughout the movement. Repeat.

TRAINER'S TIP: Keep your chest up to prevent the weights pulling your shoulders forward.

HALFWAY THERE. REMEMBER WHY YOU'RE DOING THIS!

11. SQUAT JUMPS

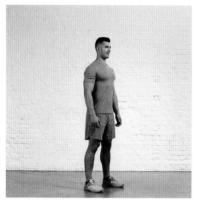

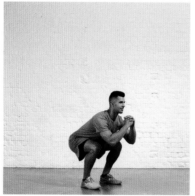

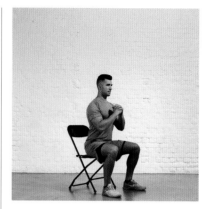

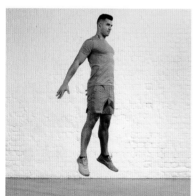

Stand with your feet shoulder-width apart. Lower your body into a squat. Jump off the floor as explosively as you can, driving your arms outward and downward. Return to the starting position and repeat.

TRAINER'S TIP: Use your arms to drive the movement up and power up by placing the force in your heels, and really push the ground away with your feet.

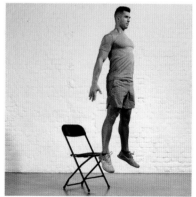

BEGINNERS: If you struggle with the impact of jumping, try sitting down on a chair and standing up as explosively as you can, working up to jumping up off the chair.

SQUAT TILL YOU DROP AND GET THAT ASS TO THE GRASS!

12. LEFT LEG RUNNER'S LUNGE

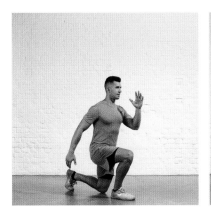 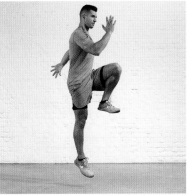 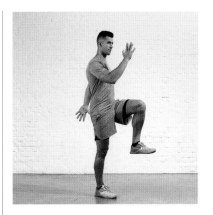

Stand with your feet hip-width apart. Step your left foot back, tapping the left knee to the floor, and raise your left hand up toward your face. Then drive your left knee high to your chest, jumping your right foot off the floor, swinging your left arm back and your right arm forward. Repeat on this side only.

TRAINER'S TIP: Use your arms as a counterbalance, as you would if you were running, to steady you.

BEGINNERS: If you cannot jump, drive through with the left leg, but do not jump off the floor with the right.

13. RIGHT LEG RUNNER'S LUNGE

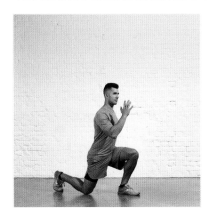 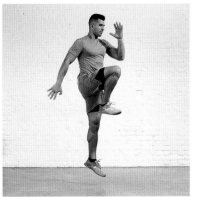 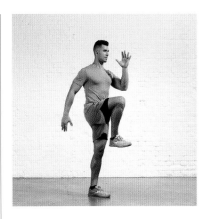

Follow the instructions for Left Leg Runner's Lunge, switching sides – step your right foot back, then drive it forwards, and jump your left foot off the floor.

TRAINER'S TIP: Keep your chest high – don't be tempted to lean your upper body down as you lunge back.

BEGINNERS: If you cannot jump, drive through with the right leg but do not jump off the floor with the left.

14. DROP SQUATS

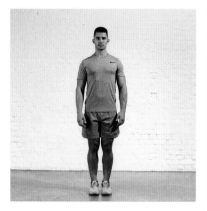 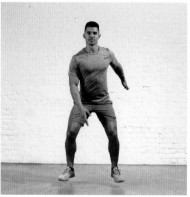 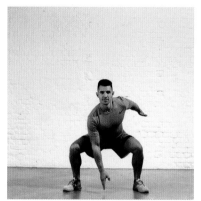

Stand with your feet close together, then jump them outward to drop into a squat. Jump your feet back in together to return to standing. Repeat.

TRAINER'S TIP: Use your hands to touch the floor between your legs, alternating sides, to encourage a deep squat.

---

15. LUNGE JUMPS

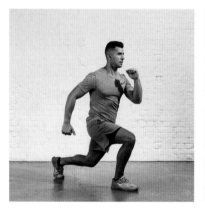 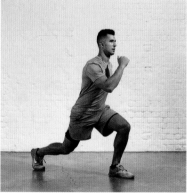

Stand with your feet hip-width apart. Step forward with your right foot and lower your hips to bring your left knee toward the floor. Drive the weight down through your right heel as you push back up, to jump directly into a lunge on the opposite side. Repeat, jumping between left and right leg lunges.

TRAINER'S TIP: Always look forward when you lunge, and use your arms in a running motion as a counterbalance.

JUST FIVE MOVES TO GO. REMEMBER, HEALTH IS WEALTH, SO KEEP PUSHING!

16. DUMBBELL SUMO SQUATS

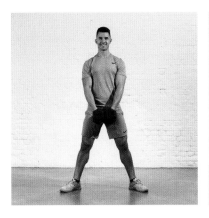 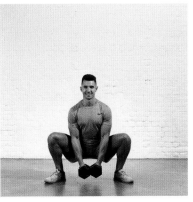 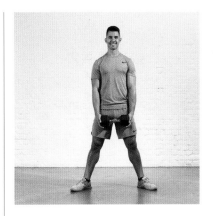

Stand with your feet slightly wider than shoulder-width apart and your toes and knees angled outward. Hold both weights by your groin. Bend your knees and squat the weights down to the floor, then return to standing. Repeat.

TRAINER'S TIP: Keep your arms extended at all times.

BEGINNERS: Use one weight, holding it with both hands.

17. DUMBBELL REVERSE LUNGES

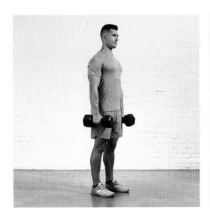 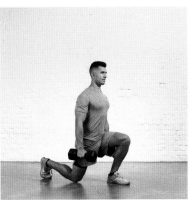 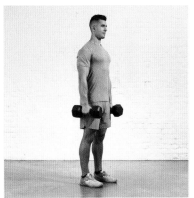

Stand with your feet shoulder-width apart and hold your weights by your sides. Step back with your right foot into a lunge, bringing your right knee toward the floor, then return to standing. Repeat, alternating legs.

TRAINER'S TIP: Keep looking forward and focus on getting your back knee as close to the floor as possible.

18. DUMBBELL SWING SQUATS

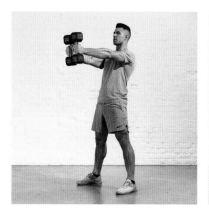 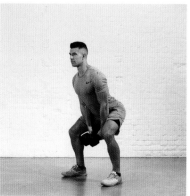 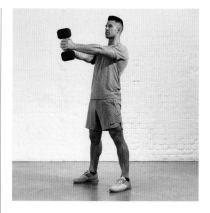

Stand with your feet slightly wider than shoulder-width apart. Touch both weights together in front of you, with arms straight and palms facing each other. Hinging at the hip, bend your knees and push your bum back, then thrust your hips forward, creating a swinging motion with the weights to raise them up in front of you. Reverse then repeat the move to keep the momentum of the swing going for 40 seconds.

BEGINNERS: Try it with just one weight.

TRAINER'S TIP: Don't expect the weights to swing higher than your eye line – the thrusting strength of the hips won't have enough momentum to power them further.

19. DUMBBELL FRONT KICKS

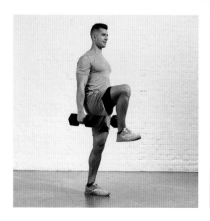 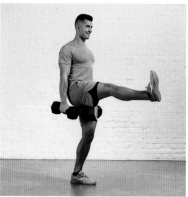 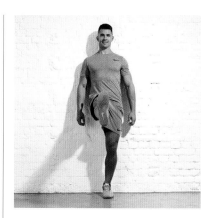

Stand with your feet together, holding your weights in your hands by your sides. Bring your right knee up to a 90° angle in front of you, then straighten your right knee to kick the leg forward. Release the leg and come back to standing, then repeat, alternating legs.

TRAINER'S TIP: Keep your core tight and engaged while your chest stays high to keep your balance.

BEGINNERS: Practise this movement against a wall, without weights.

20. DUMBBELL KNEELING TO STANDING

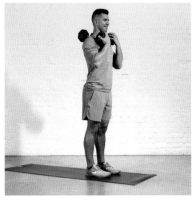
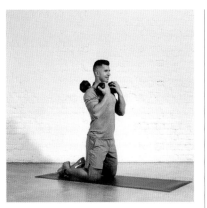
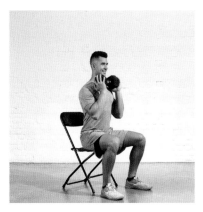

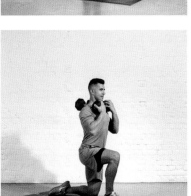
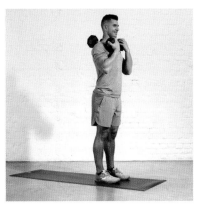
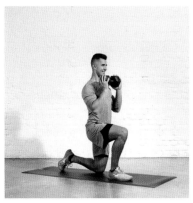

Stand with your feet together, holding a dumbbell on each shoulder as shown. Bring your right knee to the floor, then the left knee, so that you are kneeling on both knees. Step forward with your right foot and return to standing. Repeat, alternating legs.

TRAINER'S TIP: Use a mat or folded towel under you to lessen the impact when you kneel. Keep upright, with a flat back.

BEGINNERS: If kneeling is too hard, try standing from a sitting position on a chair or sofa, or use just one weight to lessen the load.

NOW TURN TO MY COOL-DOWN RECOVERY SEQUENCE ON PAGES 122–7.

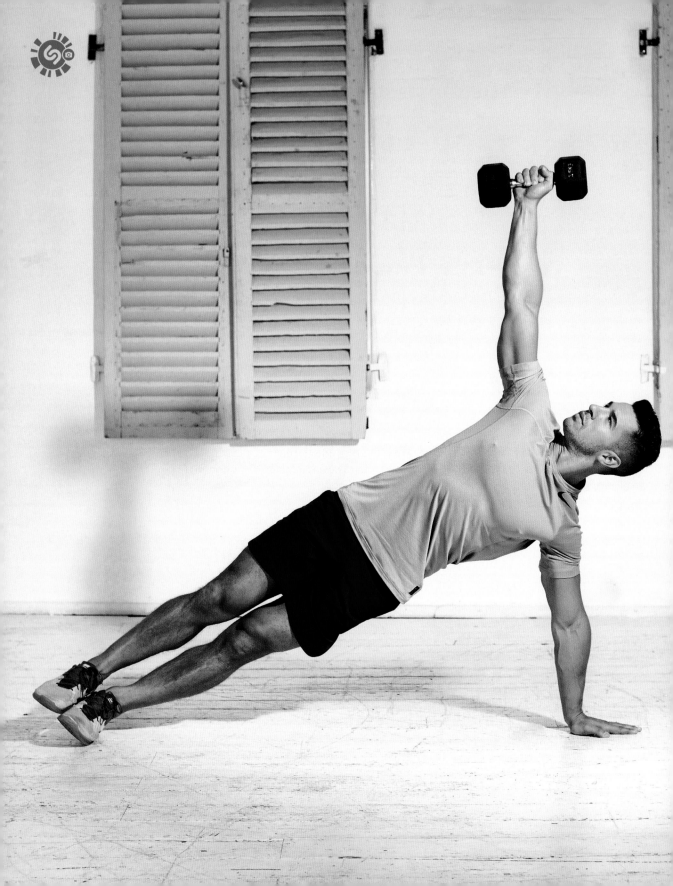

WEEK ONE
DAY THREE/WEDNESDAY
CHEST, BACK AND CORE

1. T-ROTATION

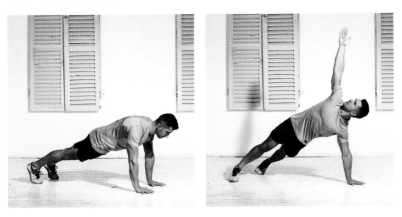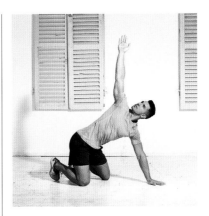

Get into plank position. With your right hand, reach out to the side and up toward the ceiling to open up your chest. Bring the arm back down and return to plank position, then repeat, alternating arms.

TRAINER'S TIP: Follow your hand with your eyes to ensure full rotation. Keep your hands beneath your shoulders when in plank.

BEGINNERS: Drop to your knees and perform the same movement.

2. SUPERMAN/SUPERWOMAN

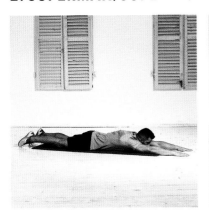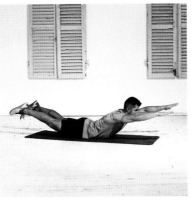

Lie face-down on the floor with your arms and legs fully extended. From this starting position, raise your chest and hips off the floor, keeping your arms and legs straight. Return to the starting position, then repeat.

TRAINER'S TIP: Keep your eyes on the floor to keep a neutral spine. Don't strain your neck by craning it as you raise your chest.

3. PLANK

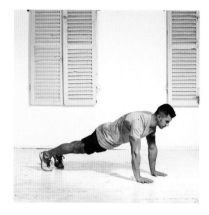
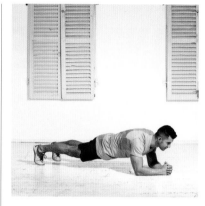

Hold a plank position for 40 seconds.

TRAINER'S TIP: Keep your shoulders and elbows above your wrists.

BEGINNERS: Move it down to an elbow plank and balance on your elbows and forearms as you clasp your fingers together.

4. PLANK HIP TOUCH

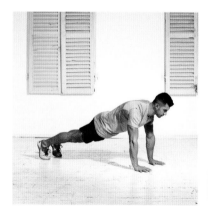
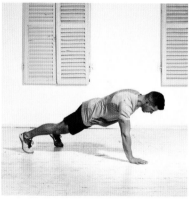
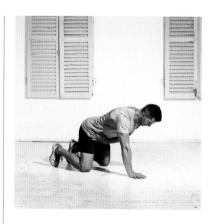

Get into plank position. Touch your right hip with left hand, then return to plank position. Repeat, alternating arms and sides.

TRAINER'S TIP: Keep your feet shoulder-width apart for balance and concentrate on keeping your hips parallel to the floor so they don't rock or raise with the hip-reaching movement.

BEGINNERS: Drop to your knees to perform the movement.

5. PUSH UP TO REACH

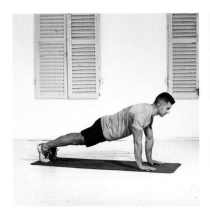 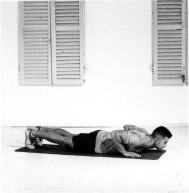 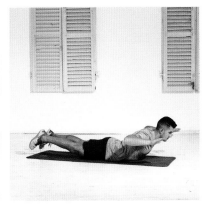

Get into plank position. Bend your elbows to lower your body toward the floor. Raise your arms out to the sides, elbows bent. Raise your chest off the ground and then return your hands back under your shoulders and push the floor away from you to return to a plank position.

TRAINER'S TIP: Perform this movement slowly to experience the full range of movement.

6. DUMBBELL CHEST PRESS – PRONATED GRIP

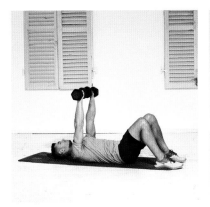 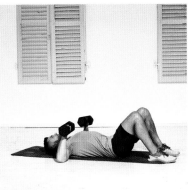 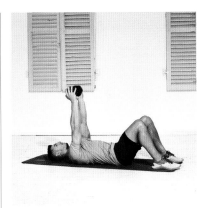

Lie on your back with your knees bent and your feet flat on the floor. Hold a weight in each hand with your palms facing toward your feet, and your elbows on the floor. Fully extend your arms upward above you, keeping the palms facing away from you. From this starting position, bend your elbows and lower them out to the sides and down to the floor. They should tap the floor before you press back up to the starting position. Repeat.

TRAINER'S TIP: Breathe out when you press, and breathe in when you lower your elbows to the floor.

BEGINNERS: Hold one weight with both hands by the weighted ends. Bring it down to your chest, then raise it back up.

7. DUMBBELL CLOSE GRIP PRESS

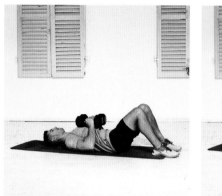 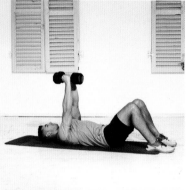 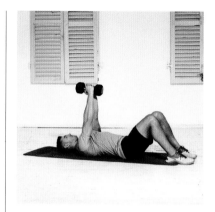

Lie on your back with your knees bent and your feet flat on the floor. Hold a weight in each hand over your chest with your palms facing each other, elbows on the floor by your sides. Fully extend your arms above your chest. Next, lower the weights to your chest, keeping your elbows tight to your body. Repeat.

BEGINNERS: Use one dumbbell and hold the handle with both hands, palms facing each other.

TRAINER'S TIP: Keep the weights touching at all times.

8. DUMBBELL SEE-SAW PRESS – NEUTRAL GRIP

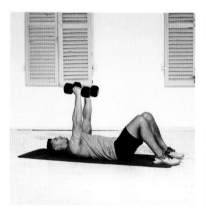 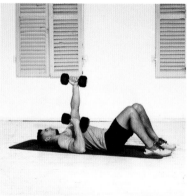 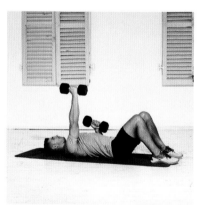

Lie on your back with your knees bent and your feet flat on the floor. Hold both weights with your wrists facing toward each other and your arms fully extended directly upward. Lower one elbow to the floor by your side. As you press this back up, lower the opposite elbow to the floor. Repeat, alternating sides in a continuous see-saw motion.

TRAINER'S TIP: If you need to stop, keep your weights raised. The floor is lava! Don't let the weights touch the floor.

9. DUMBBELL CIRCULAR CHEST PRESS

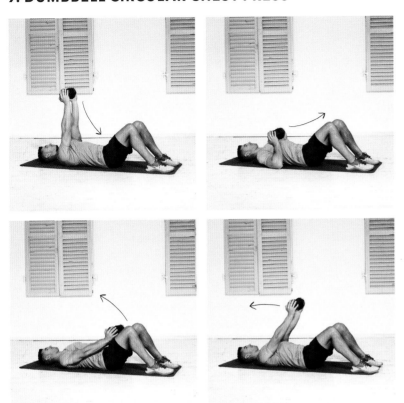

WHEN IT STARTS TO HURT, IT STARTS TO WORK SO PUSH THROUGH THAT PAIN BARRIER!

Lie on your back with your knees bent and your feet flat on the floor, holding one dumbbell with both hands by the weighted ends. Start with your arms extended above your chest. In one smooth circular movement, lower the dumbbell to your chest, travel it down your torso toward your hips, then extend your arms back to the starting position, above your chest. Repeat.

TRAINER'S TIP: Keep your elbows tight to your body and your core tight.

10. DUMBBELL OVERHEAD PULLS

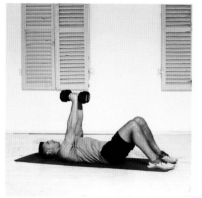 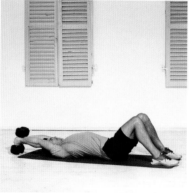 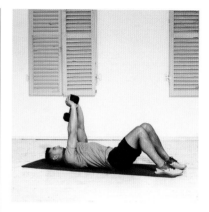

Lie on your back with your knees bent and your feet flat on the floor. Hold a weight in each hand with palms facing each other. Keeping the weights touching, extend your arms directly upward. From this starting position, keeping your arms straight, lower the weights to the floor beyond your head, brushing your ears with your upper arms. Try to touch the floor with the weights, then raise your arms back to the starting position. Repeat.

TRAINER'S TIP: Keep your arms straight and reach back as far as you can. Engage your core by keeping your back flat to the ground. If it starts to arch off the ground, you have reached your limit.

BEGINNERS: Perform the movement with one dumbbell, holding it at one end with both hands.

HALFWAY THERE! YOUR MUSCLES SHOULD BE ON FIRE NOW, BUT REMEMBER THAT NOTHING WORTH HAVING COMES EASY.

11. LEFT ARM SIDE PLANK DIPS

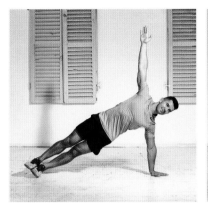 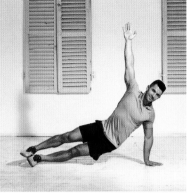 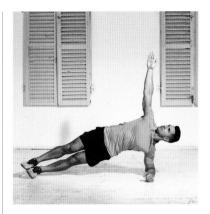

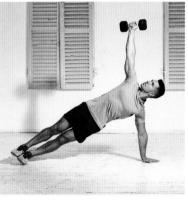

Hold a side plank on your left side with your left arm locked out. Now dip your left hip to the floor, then raise it back up to the starting position. Repeat.

TRAINER'S TIP: Either stack your feet on top of each other or place one in front of the other. Just dip your left hip – do not let your body twist.

12. REVERSE PLANK HOLD

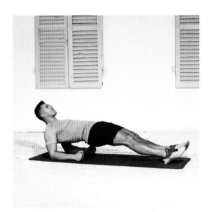
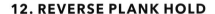

BEGINNERS: Do this on your elbow, or just hold the side plank position without the dips.

ADVANCED: Perform the movement with one dumbbell, holding it in your raised hand.

Lying on your back, raise up on your lower arms and support your upper body with your elbows. Now raise your hips and lower legs up off the floor as high as you can, keeping your weight balanced on your lower arms and heels. Hold this position for 40 seconds.

TRAINER'S TIP: Squeeze your bum together super tight as though you are trying to crack an egg between the cheeks. Keep those quads tight down your thighs, to try to stop your hips dropping.

13. RIGHT ARM SIDE PLANK DIPS

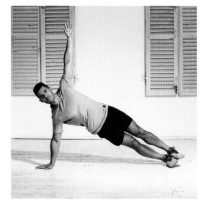 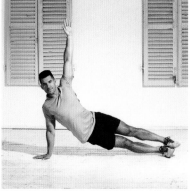 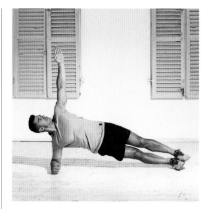

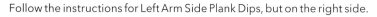

Follow the instructions for Left Arm Side Plank Dips, but on the right side.

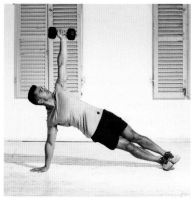

WE'RE NOT HERE TO BE AVERAGE, WE'RE HERE TO BE AWESOME. LET'S DO THIS!

BEGINNERS: Do this on your elbow, or just hold the side plank position without the dips.

ADVANCED: Perform the movement with one dumbbell, holding it in your raised hand.

14. LEFT ELBOW TO RIGHT KNEE CRUNCH

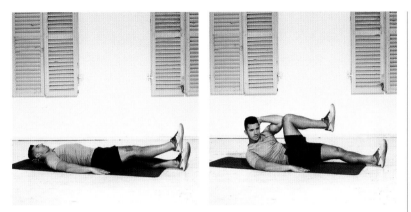

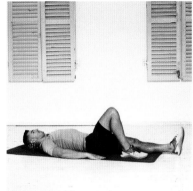

Lie on your back with your legs out flat. Place your left hand behind your head and raise your right leg slightly off the floor. As you bend your right knee to bring it toward your chest, lift your left shoulder off the floor and crunch your left elbow to meet your right knee, keeping your left leg flat on the floor. Return to the starting position, keeping your right foot off the floor, then repeat.

TRAINER'S TIP: Try to keep your right foot off the floor at all times, and crunch as much of your back up off the floor as possible. Do not use your left hand to lift your head up – use your core strength to lift yourself.

BEGINNERS: Bend your right knee and place your right foot flat on the floor. Keeping your right knee static, crunch your left elbow toward your right knee as far as you can. Return to the starting position, then repeat.

15. RIGHT ELBOW TO LEFT KNEE CRUNCH

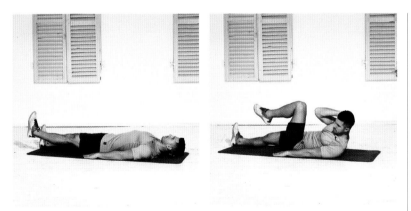

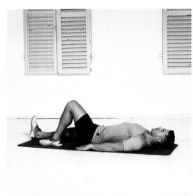

Follow the instructions for Left Elbow to Right Knee Crunch, but switching sides – crunch your right elbow to your left knee.

BEGINNERS: Follow the beginners' instructions for Left Elbow to Right Knee Crunch, but switching sides.

16. DUMBBELL DEADLIFTS

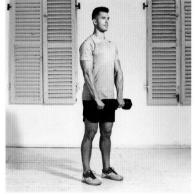 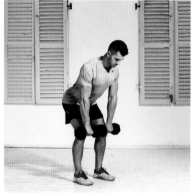 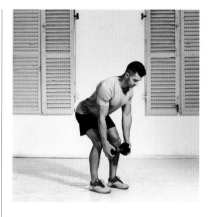

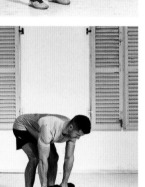

Stand with a dumbbell in each hand and hold them in front of you with your palms facing your body. Keeping your back straight, hinge at your hips, push your bum back and bend slightly at the knees to lower the dumbbells to your ankles. Unhinge your hips and, keeping the weights close to the line of your legs, raise back up to standing. Repeat.

TRAINER'S TIP: Keep your eyes focussed on the floor about 2.5cm (1 inch) in front of your feet. Keep your back flat at all times and don't arch the back by leaning back when you come back to standing.

BEGINNERS: Try this with one dumbbell.

FIVE MOVES LEFT.
HONEST TRAINING = HONEST RESULTS,
SO GIVE IT EVERYTHING YOU'VE GOT.

17. DUMBBELL HIGH PULLS

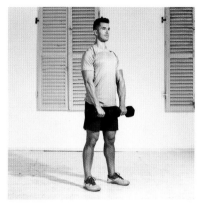 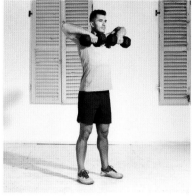 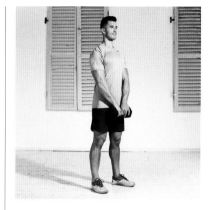

Stand tall, holding a dumbbell in each hand in front of your body, with your palms facing your body. Pull the dumbbells up to your chin and bring your elbows high, then lower them back to the starting position. Repeat.

TRAINER'S TIP: Keep the weights close to your body.

BEGINNERS: Hold one dumbbell only with both hands to perform this movement.

18. DUMBBELL BENT-OVER WIDE ROWS

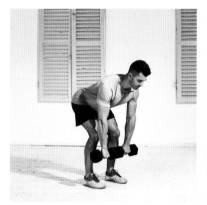 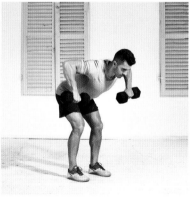 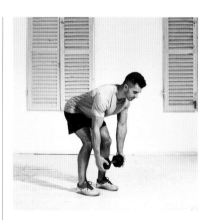

Stand in a bent-over position, with back flat and chest over your toes. Hold a dumbbell in each hand, with arms extended straight down toward the floor and your palms facing your body. From this starting position, bend your elbows out to the sides and up, to form 90° angles. Pinch your shoulder blades together. Lower your arms back to the starting position and repeat.

TRAINER'S TIP: Keep your back flat and focus on something on the floor.

BEGINNERS: Perform with one dumbbell. Hold it by either end and stand in the bent-over position, then lift the dumbbell up toward your chest. Lower your arms back to the starting position and repeat.

19. DUMBBELL RENEGADE ROWS

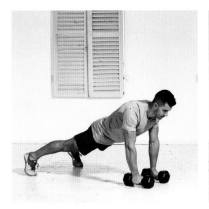 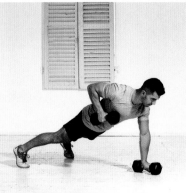 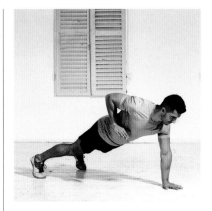

Get into plank position and hold each weight like a hammer as your base. Spread your feet out wide. Pull one dumbbell off the floor to your chest, then lower it back to the floor. Repeat, alternating arms.

TRAINER'S TIP: Keep your shoulders over your wrists and your hips parallel to the floor, so your torso doesn't twist as you rip the weight up. Really focus on keeping the hips still throughout the movement and keep your elbows tight to your body when you row the dumbbells off the floor.

BEGINNERS: Perform the movement with no dumbbells and keep one palm flat on the floor, as with a regular plank, when rowing to your chest with the opposite arm.

GET COMFORTABLE WITH BEING UNCOMFORTABLE BECAUSE THIS ISN'T SUPPOSED TO BE EASY. THE SERIOUSLY GOOD STUFF BEGINS OUTSIDE YOUR COMFORT ZONE.

20. DUMBBELL DEADLIFT TO HIGH PULL

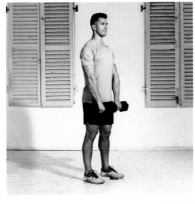
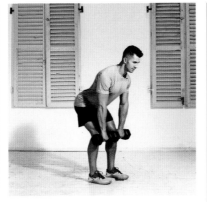
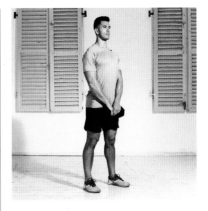

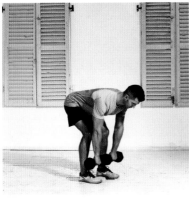
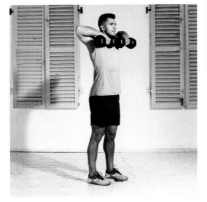

BEGINNERS: Perform the movement with one weight, holding it by the handle in both hands.

Stand holding your dumbbells in front of your body, with your palms facing your body. From this starting position, keeping your back straight, hinge at your hips and bend slightly at the knees to lower the dumbbells to your ankles. Keeping the slight bend in your knees, unhinge back up through your hips to return to standing. From here, pull the dumbbells up to your chin, bringing your elbows out high, and then lower them to the starting position. Repeat the entire sequence.

TRAINER'S TIP: Don't rush. Take your time and remember to look at the floor when you deadlift and to look straight ahead when you high pull.

TURN TO MY COOL-DOWN RECOVERY SEQUENCE ON PAGES 122–7.

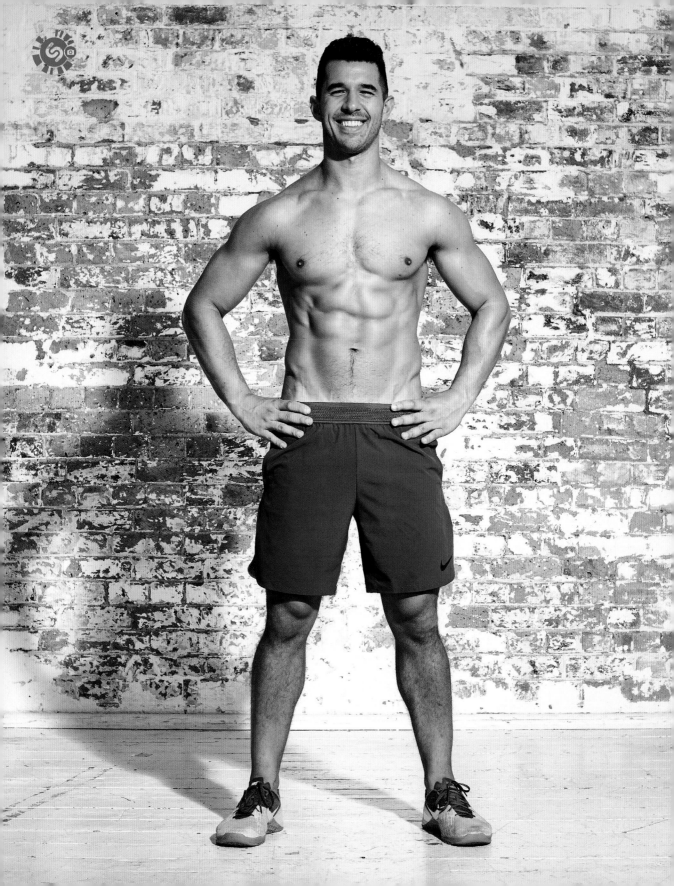

WEEK ONE
DAY FOUR/THURSDAY

ABS AND CORE

1. STANDING KNEE CRUNCH

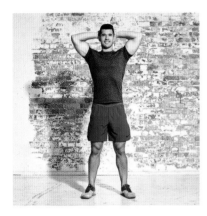 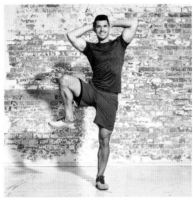 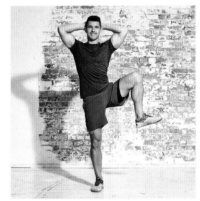

Stand with your feet shoulder-width apart and with your hands held behind your head. Raise and crunch your right knee out toward your right elbow, then lower it back to standing. Repeat, alternating sides.

TRAINER'S TIP: Concentrate on crunching your knee outside your body rather than in front of it. Try to bring your knee to your elbow, rather than your elbow to your knee. Keep your hips facing forwards – don't twist.

IT DOESN'T GET EASIER,
BUT YOU WILL GET BETTER!

2. HIGH KNEES

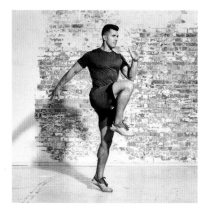 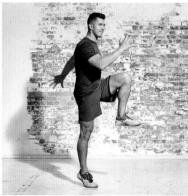

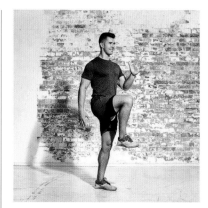

Stand with your feet hip-width apart and run on the spot, raising your knees as high as possible when you do so.

TRAINER'S TIP: Use your arms to drive and pump the action to get your knees as high as possible.

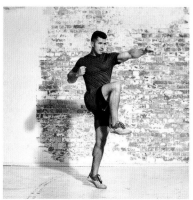

LOOK IN THE MIRROR; THAT'S YOUR COMPETITION. LOOK YOURSELF IN THE EYE AND DARE YOURSELF TO SMASH OUT THE BEST WORKOUT YOU'VE EVER DONE.

BEGINNERS: Just raise your knees as high as you can without the running action, alternating sides.

ADVANCED: Take it up a level by adding in some punches as you run on the spot.

3. STAR JUMPS

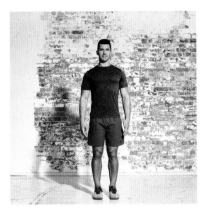 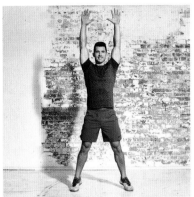 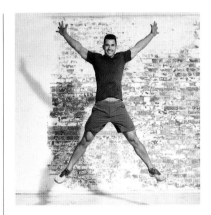

Stand with your feet together and arms by your sides. Jump both your feet out wide and raise your arms up above your head, then outward, landing in a star shape. Jump your feet back in and land with your arms back at your sides. Repeat.

TRAINER'S TIP: Think big. Make the action exaggerated to experience a full range of motion.

ADVANCED: Make the star jump one continuous movement – as you jump, stretch out your arms and legs to form the star shape at the height of the movement, then land with your feet together and your arms by your side. Make the movements into and out of the star shape explosive.

4. PLANK JUMPING JACKS

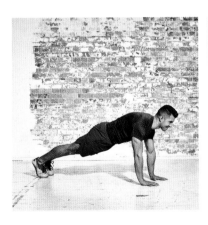 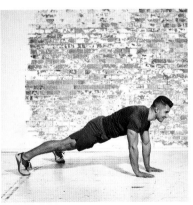

Get into plank position with your feet together. Jump your feet out wide, then jump them back together. Repeat.

TRAINER'S TIP: No bums in the air! Keep your hips low at all times, and your shoulders over your wrists.

5. TWISTING MOUNTAIN CLIMBERS

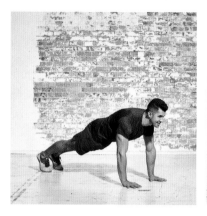 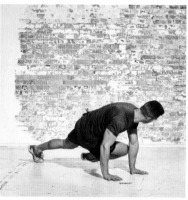 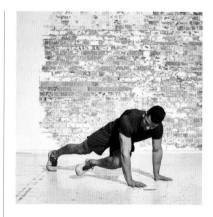

Get into plank position with your feet hip-width apart. Take your right foot off the floor, crunch your right knee toward your left elbow, then return to plank. Repeat, alternating legs and sides.

TRAINER'S TIP: Keep your shoulders over your wrists to stop your body from rocking forward.

ADVANCED: Pick up the pace and do this quick time, but be careful not to lose form on your plank. Technique is always better than speed.

6. PLANK TUCKS

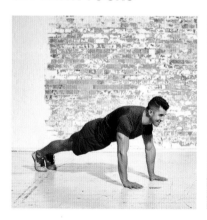 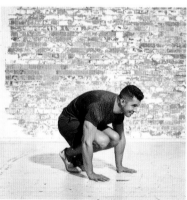 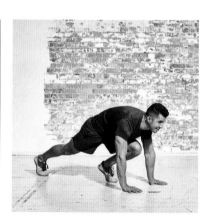

Get into plank position, with your feet together. Jump your feet in toward your chest, then back to plank. Repeat.

TRAINER'S TIP: Finding your rhythm with this continuous movement will help you stay strong.

BEGINNERS: Step your feet in toward your chest one at a time, then step back into plank.

7. LEFT SIDE PLANK HOLD

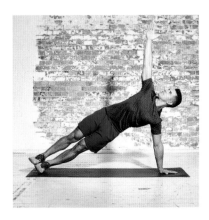

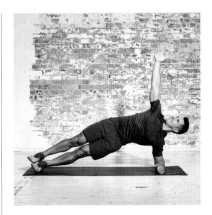

Get into a side plank on your left side with your right arm extended upward. Hold for 40 seconds.

TRAINER'S TIP: Stack your feet or place them one in front of the other.

BEGINNERS: Drop down onto your left elbow and hold an elbow side plank.

8. ELBOW PLANK

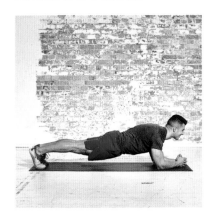

WHAT IS YOUR WHY? WHY ARE YOU DOING THIS? WHY ARE YOU PUTTING YOURSELF THROUGH THIS? REMEMBER WHY YOU WANT IT AND DON'T YOU DARE QUIT ON ME!

Get into an elbow plank, with your eyes focussed on a point on the floor. Hold for 40 seconds.

TRAINER'S TIP: Really squeeze your glutes.

9. RIGHT SIDE PLANK HOLD

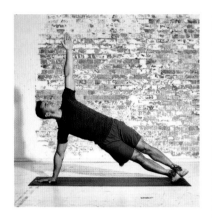 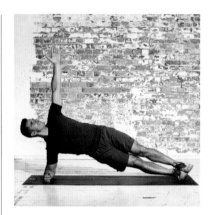

Get into a side plank on your right side with your left arm extended upward. Hold for 40 seconds.

TRAINER'S TIP: Stack your feet one on top of the other, or place them one in front of the other.

BEGINNERS: Drop down onto your right elbow and hold an elbow side plank.

10. PLANK SEE-SAW

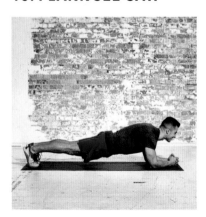 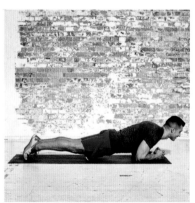

Get into an elbow plank position with your feet together. Rock your body forward, taking your shoulders past your elbows, and then rock back to the original elbow plank position. Repeat.

TRAINER'S TIP: Flex your ankles as you rock back to allow a further reach.

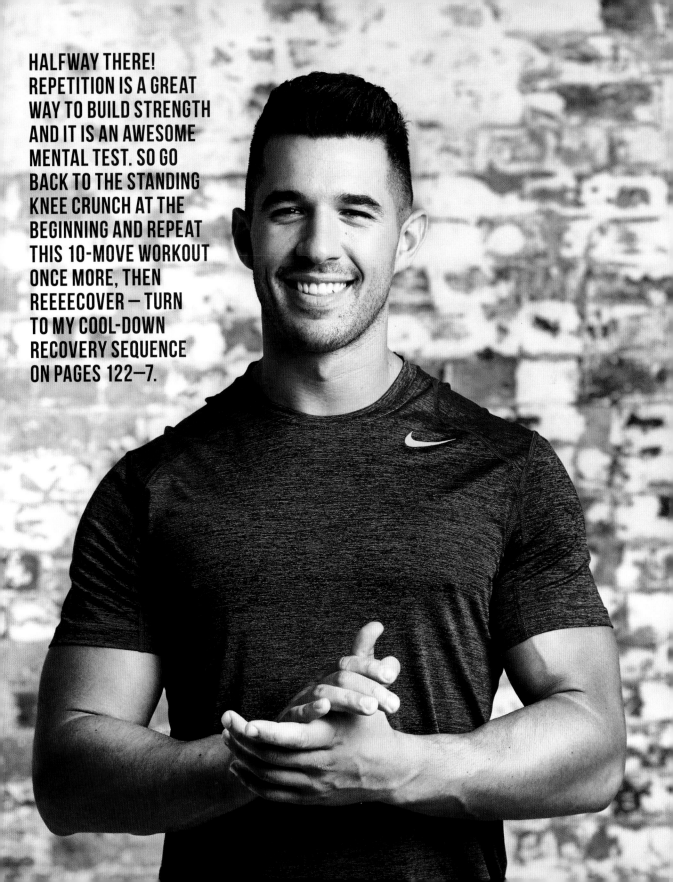

HALFWAY THERE! REPETITION IS A GREAT WAY TO BUILD STRENGTH AND IT IS AN AWESOME MENTAL TEST. SO GO BACK TO THE STANDING KNEE CRUNCH AT THE BEGINNING AND REPEAT THIS 10-MOVE WORKOUT ONCE MORE, THEN REEEECOVER — TURN TO MY COOL-DOWN RECOVERY SEQUENCE ON PAGES 122–7.

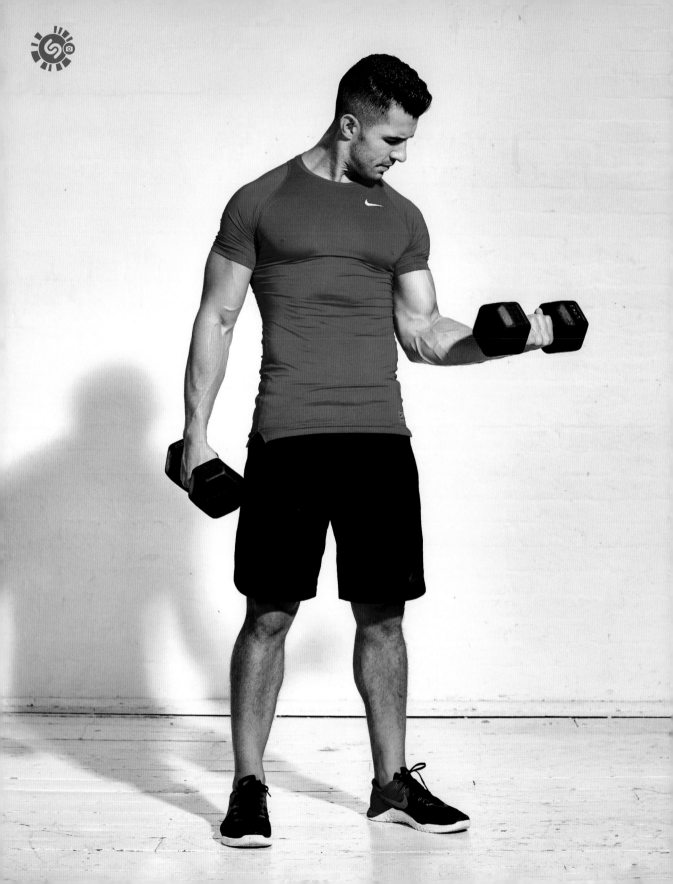

WEEK ONE
DAY FIVE/FRIDAY
FULL BODY WITH WEIGHTS

1. WALKOUTS

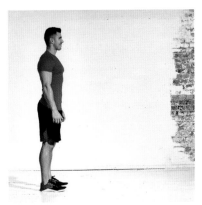
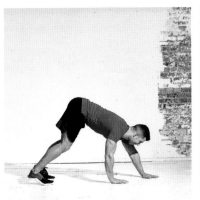
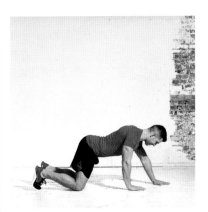

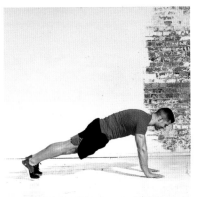
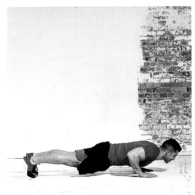

Begin in a standing position. Bend forward at the hips, keeping your legs as straight as possible, and rest your hands on the floor below your shoulders. Now walk your hands out in front of you into push up position. Walk your hands back beneath your shoulders, then uncurl your back one vertebra at a time as you come up to standing. Repeat.

TRAINER'S TIP: Try to keep your legs straight at all times.

BEGINNERS: Walk out from a kneeling position. Start in a kneeling position with your hands on the floor in front of your knees. Walk your hands out to an all-fours position, then back again to the starting position.

ADVANCED: Add in a press up when you get to your plank position before walking back up.

2. PLANK

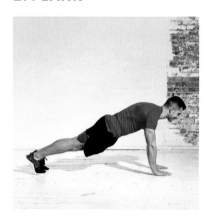

Hold a high plank position for 40 seconds.

TRAINER'S TIP: Squeeze your glutes tight as though you are holding a pencil between your bum cheeks, and really try to push your hands into the floor.

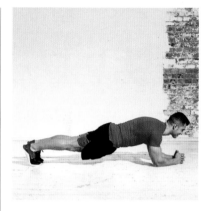

BEGINNERS: Hold an elbow plank.

3. PUSH-UPS

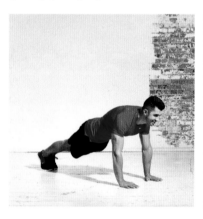
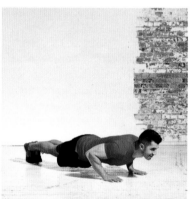
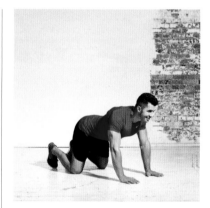
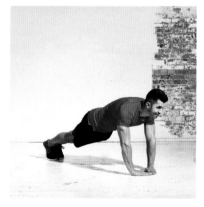

Hold a plank position with your feet together. Bend your elbows, keeping them tucked into the body, to lower your chest to the floor, then push up back to plank. Repeat.

TRAINER'S TIP: Always kiss your chest to the floor and look down. It is better to perform a few push ups well than do lots of "half reps".

BEGINNERS: Drop to your knees for your push-ups, but ensure you are still kissing your chest to the floor.

ADVANCED: Move your hands closer together to make this move even more challenging.

4. ELBOW PLANK

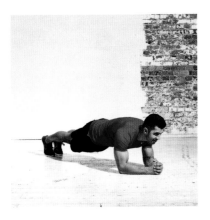

Get into an elbow plank, keeping your core tight and your body straight. Hold for 40 seconds.

TRAINER'S TIP: Keep your shoulders over your elbows and squeeze your glutes in.

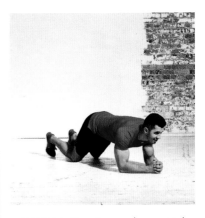

BEGINNERS: Drop to your knees and hold an elbow plank.

5. PIKE PUSH-UPS

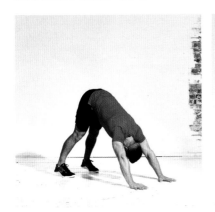
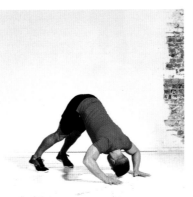
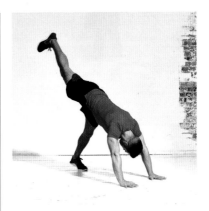

Get into a pike position, with your feet hip-width apart, hips up in the air and your head between your shoulders. From this starting position, bend your elbows, lower the top of your head to the floor, then straighten your elbows as though you are performing a push-up to return to the starting position. Repeat.

TRAINER'S TIP: Keep your hips up as high as possible and look at your toes.

ADVANCED: Raise your right leg off the floor when you straighten your arms. Hold for 20 seconds, then repeat, alternating sides.

6. DUMBBELL SQUAT CURLS

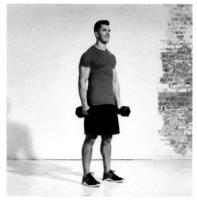 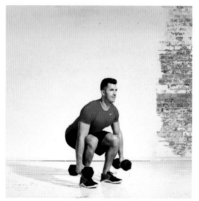 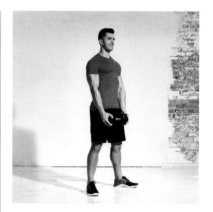

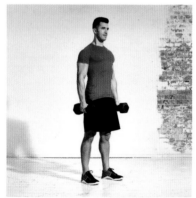 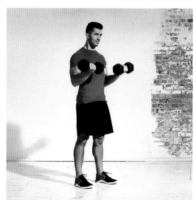

BEGINNERS: Stand holding one dumbbell by each weighted end in front of you. Squat with your knees outside your arms, return to standing, then curl the dumbbell up to your shoulders. Return to standing, then repeat.

Stand with your feet shoulder-width apart, holding a dumbbell in each hand by your sides. Bend your knees at a 90° angle into a squat, keeping your arms outside your knees, then return to standing. When back in the standing position, curl the dumbbells up to your shoulders with your palms facing up, then return them to your sides. Repeat.

TRAINER'S TIP: Keep your chest up and back straight throughout. Elbows should remain tight into the sides of your body when performing the dumbbell curl.

DON'T FORGET THAT YOU'RE DOING THIS FOR YOU. KEEP PUSHING, KEEP DRIVING AND LET'S GET YOU TO THE BEST VERSION OF YOU.

7. DUMBBELL SQUAT TRICEP EXTENSION

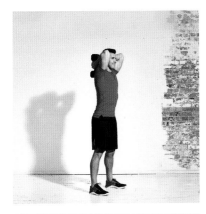
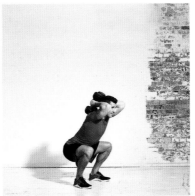
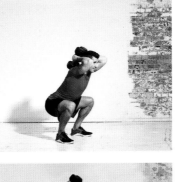
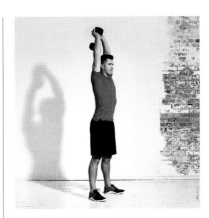
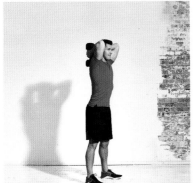
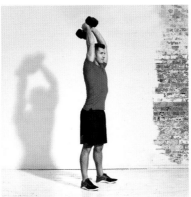

BEGINNERS: Perform this movement holding an end of one dumbbell with both hands.

Stand holding your weights in your hands behind your head, with your elbows bent and pointing up. From this starting position, squat down, bending your knees at 90° angles, then return to standing. From standing, straighten your elbows to extend the dumbbells above your head, then lower them back to the starting position. Repeat.

TRAINER'S TIP: Keep your elbows tucked tightly into your head when squatting, and keep your core engaged. The easiest way to engage your core is to imagine you are about to be punched in the stomach. You'd instinctively contract your abs to protect yourself.

8. DUMBBELL SQUAT PRESS

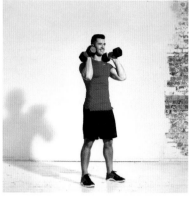 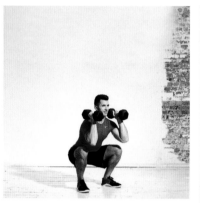 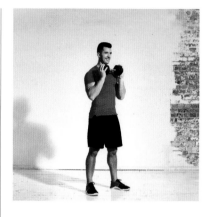

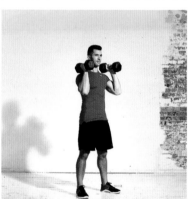 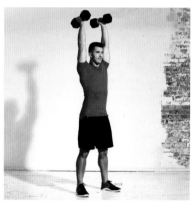

BEGINNERS: Hold one weight by each weighted end and tuck it under your chin as you squat.

Stand with your feet shoulder-width apart and hold your weights at your shoulders as shown. Squat down, bending your knees to form a 90° angle, then return to standing. Next, straighten your elbows to press the weights above your head, then lower them back to your shoulders. Repeat.

TRAINER'S TIP: Keep your back flat and your chest up. If you need a little help getting the weights up on the press, bend your knees slightly and use them to add a push to the action.

9. DUMBBELL SHOULDER T-RAISES

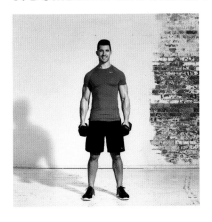
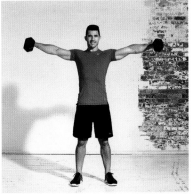

Stand with your feet shoulder-width apart and hold a weight in each hand by your sides. Raise both arms straight out to the sides, to shoulder height (your palms should be facing the floor), then lower them back to the starting position. Repeat.

TRAINER'S TIP: Keep your core engaged and control the weights. This movement is not about speed.

BEGINNERS: Perform without weights.

10. DUMBBELL LUNGE BICEP CURLS

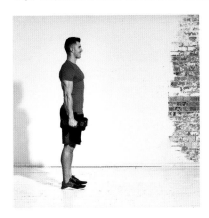
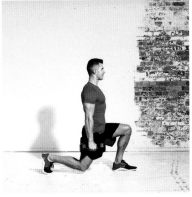
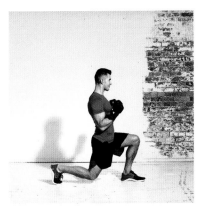

Stand with your feet hip-width apart and hold one weight in each hand by your sides, palms facing inward. Step forward with your left foot, bend your knees and bring your right knee to the floor – each knee should form a 90° angle. Hold this lunge position as you curl the dumbbells up to your shoulders, then back down to your sides. Step your left foot back to the starting position. Repeat with the right leg leading, then repeat, alternating legs.

TRAINER'S TIP: Keep your chest up and your elbows tucked into your body when curling.

BEGINNERS: Perform without weights.

HALFWAY THERE. THE SWEAT SHOULD BE DRIPPING BY NOW, BUT YOU NEED TO TRAIN LIKE A BEAST TO FEEL LIKE A BEAUTY, AS THEY SAY.

11. DUMBBELL OVERHEAD LUNGES

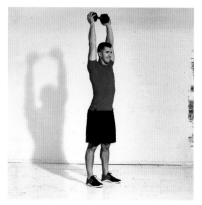 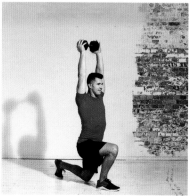

Stand with your feet hip-width apart and hold a dumbbell by the weighted ends with your arms raised straight up to hold the weight above your head. From this starting position, step forward with your right foot, bend your knees and bring your left knee to the floor – each knee should form a 90° angle. Step the right foot back and return to standing, keeping the weight held high. Now lunge on the other side – step forward with the left foot and bring your right knee to the floor. Return to standing, keeping the weight held high, and repeat.

TRAINER'S TIP: Keep looking forward and focus on engaging your core.

ADVANCED: Perform the move with two weights, holding them in your hands with the palms facing each other.

KEEP PUSHING. LET'S GET HUNGRY FOR IT AND FINISH WITH THAT TANK EMPTY. HOLDING STUFF BACK IN RESERVE IS A WASTE OF YOUR TIME AND MINE, SO GIVE EVERYTHING YOU'VE GOT!

12. DUMBBELL LEFT LEG DEADLIFT TO ROW

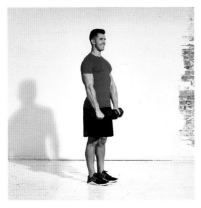 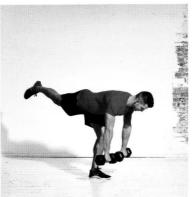 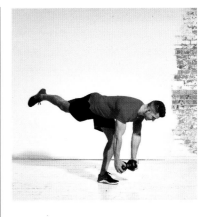

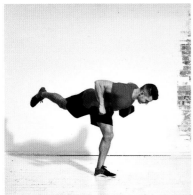 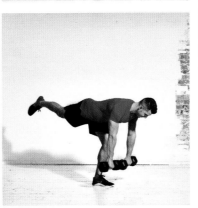

BEGINNERS: Perform this exercise holding just one weight by the weighted ends in your hands, or without weights.

Stand with your feet together and the weights in your hands by your sides, with palms facing backward. Hinging at the hips, raise your right leg behind you and settle your weight into your left leg. Aim to keep your right leg straight and your heel pointing toward the ceiling. Bend forward so your chest is over your toes. Hold for a few seconds. Now row your weights up to your shoulders, with your elbows moving up toward the sky and your shoulder blades pinching together. Straighten your arms to lower the weights, bring your right leg to the floor and return to standing. Repeat.

TRAINER'S TIP: Keep your mind on your left toes for balance, keep your back flat and control the movement, focusing on balance and technique rather than speed.

13. DUMBBELL RIGHT LEG DEADLIFT TO CURL

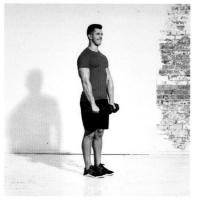 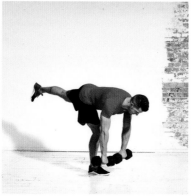 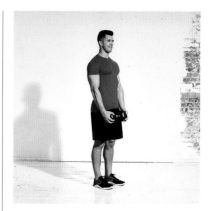

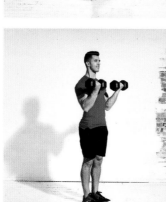

BEGINNERS: Perform this exercise holding just one weight by the weighted ends in your hands, or without weights.

Stand with your feet together and the weights in your hands by your sides, with palms facing backward. Hinging at the hips, raise your left leg behind you and settle your weight into your right leg. Aim to keep your left leg straight and your heel pointing toward the ceiling. Bend forward so your chest is over your toes. Hold for a few seconds, then return to standing. When back in the standing position, curl the dumbbells up to your shoulders with your palms facing up, then return them to your sides. Repeat.

TRAINER'S TIP: Try to keep your left foot off the floor at all times and just hover it above the ground when you return to standing. Keep your back flat and your core engaged.

14. DUMBBELL FROG SQUATS

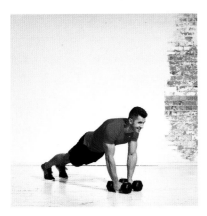 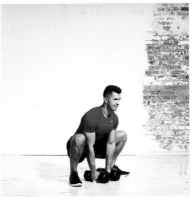 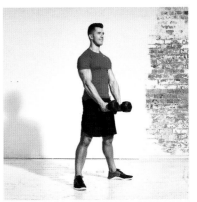

Get into plank position and hold each weight like a hammer as your base. Either step or jump your feet in to land outside each dumbbell. Bring your chest up and straighten your knees to move to standing. Lower your weights back to the floor, then jump or step your feet back to plank position. Repeat.

TRAINER'S TIP: Make sure your back is straight before you stand up, so that your lower back does not take the strain of lifting the weights. The drive should come from your legs.

BEGINNERS: Perform this move with no weights and bring your feet as far toward your hands as you can, depending on your flexibility.

15. DUMBBELL WOOD CHOPS

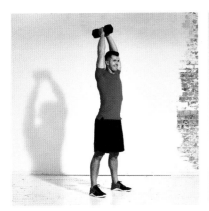 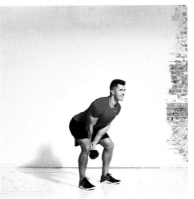 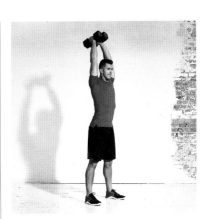

Stand with feet shoulder-width apart, holding one weight in front of you. Raise your arms above your head, then bend your knees and swing the weight down between your knees in a chopping action. Swing the weight back above your head and return to standing. Repeat in a continuous swinging motion.

TRAINER'S TIP: Keep your back flat and use your hips to create the movement.

BEGINNERS: Perform with no weights.

ADVANCED: Perform holding a weight in each hand.

JUST FIVE MOVES LEFT. DO YOU WANT TO FINISH THIS STRONG, OR LIMP ACROSS THE FINISH LINE?

16. PIKE PUSH-UPS

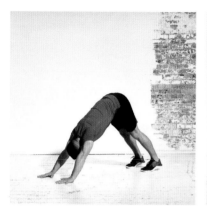 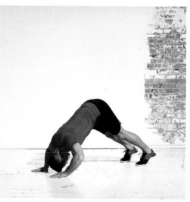

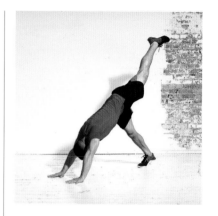

Get into a pike position, with your feet hip-width apart, hips up in the air and your head between your shoulders. From this starting position, bend your elbows, lower the top of your head to floor, then straighten your elbows as though you are performing a push-up to return to the starting position. Repeat.

TRAINER'S TIP: Keep your hips up as high as possible and look at your toes.

ADVANCED: Raise your left leg off the floor when you straighten your arms. Hold for 20 seconds, then repeat, alternating sides.

17. ELBOW PLANK

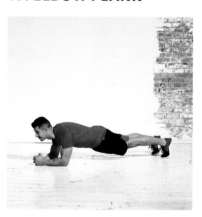

Rest on your elbows and hold a plank position for 40 seconds.

TRAINER'S TIP: Keep your shoulders over your elbows and squeeze your glutes in tight.

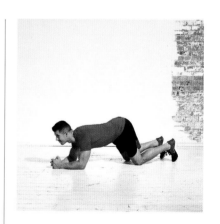

BEGINNERS: Drop to your knees.

18. PUSH-UPS

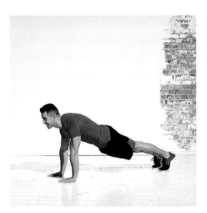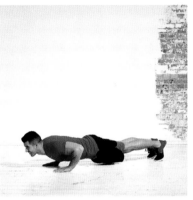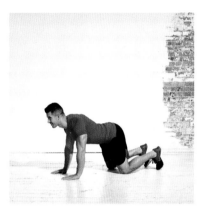

Get into plank position with your feet together. Lower your chest to the floor, then push up back to plank. Repeat.

TRAINER'S TIP: Always kiss your chest to the floor and look down.

BEGINNERS: Drop to your knees and do your push ups, but ensure you still kiss your chest to the floor.

19. PLANK

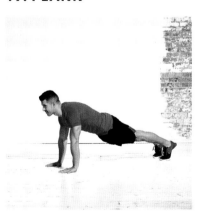

Hold a plank position for 40 seconds.

TRAINER'S TIP: Squeeze your glutes tight, as though you are holding a pencil between your bum cheeks, and push your hands into the floor.

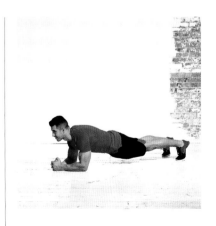

BEGINNERS: Hold an elbow plank.

20. WALKOUTS

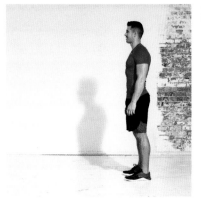 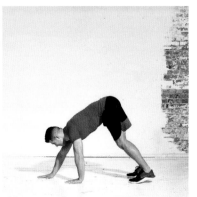 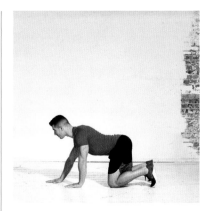

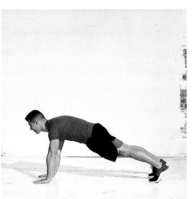 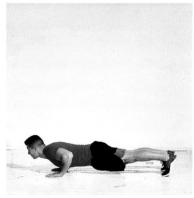

Begin in a standing position. Bend forward at the hips, keeping your legs as straight as possible, and rest your hands on the floor below your shoulders. Now walk your hands out in front of you into push up position. Walk your hands back to beneath your shoulders, then uncurl your back one vertebra at a time as you come up to standing. Repeat.

TRAINER'S TIP: Try to keep your legs straight.

BEGINNERS: Walk out from a kneeling position. Start in a kneeling position with your hands on the floor and walk your hands out to an all-fours position, then walk them back again.

ADVANCED: Add in a press up when you get to your plank position before walking back up.

TURN TO MY COOL-DOWN RECOVERY SEQUENCE ON PAGES 122–7.

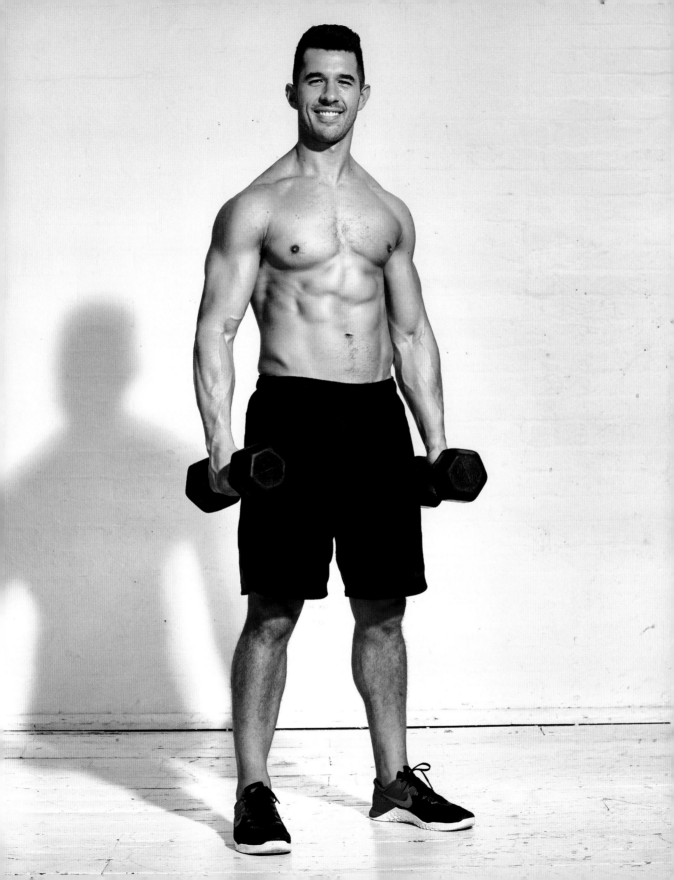

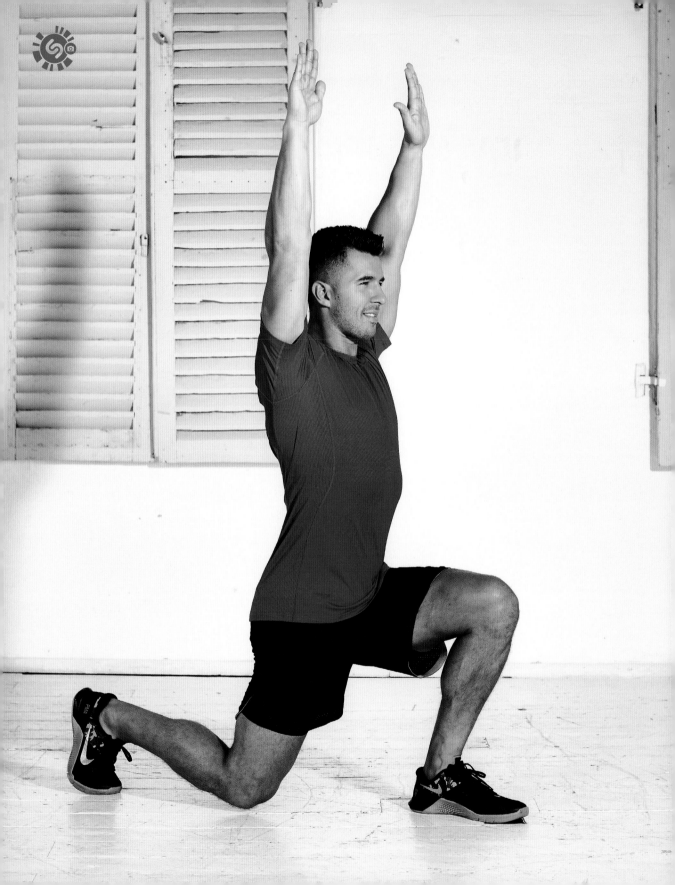

WEEK ONE
DAY SIX/SATURDAY
FULL BODY, NO WEIGHTS

1. QUICK FEET

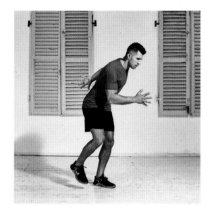
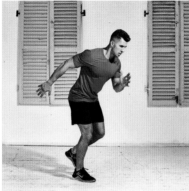

Stand with your feet shoulder-width apart. Lift your right foot behind you a little and tap your toes to the floor. Return to standing, then immediately repeat with the left foot. Repeat.

TRAINER'S TIP: Keep your upper body as still as possible. Use your arms to counter your weight as you shift from foot to foot.

2. HIGH KNEE PUNCHES

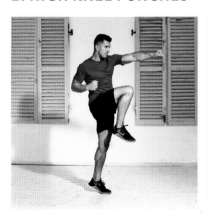
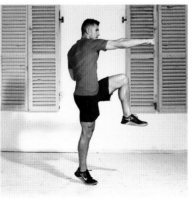
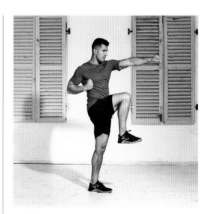

Stand with your feet hip-width apart. Run on the spot, raising your knees as high as possible. While running, punch directly in front of you with the opposite arm to the raised knee. Repeat, alternating sides.

TRAINER'S TIP: Use the opposite-arm-to-knee position to help your balance. Keep your knees high and your punches at shoulder height.

BEGINNERS: Just raise your knees as high as you can in turn, without the running action.

ADVANCED: To test your balance, try this with your eyes shut.

3. SQUAT PUNCHES

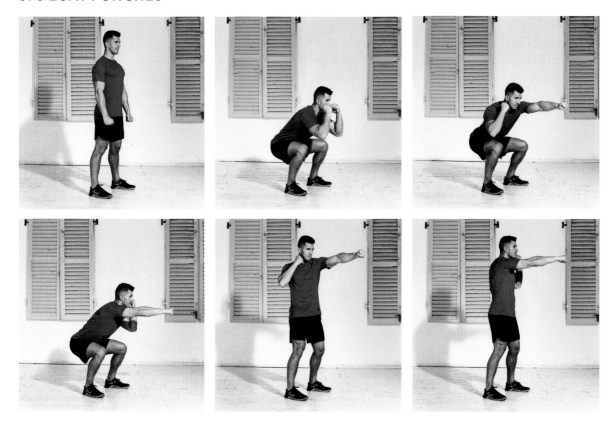

Stand with your feet shoulder-width apart. Squat low and raise your fists in front of you, ready to punch. Punch each arm in front of you once while in the squat. Come back to standing and punch each arm again. Repeat.

TRAINER'S TIP: Keep your chest high and your punches at shoulder height.

ADVANCED: Increase the number of punches to four or six each time.

DIG DEEP NOW. MAKE SURE THAT, WHEN YOU FINISH THIS, YOU CAN SAY YOU GAVE IT EVERYTHING. IF YOU CAN WORK HARDER, NOW IS THE TIME TO STEP IT UP!

4. LATERAL JUMPS

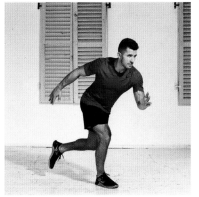 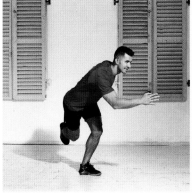 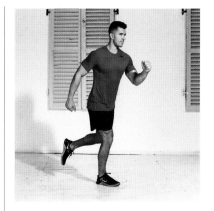

Stand with your feet together. Jump to the side on your right foot, raising your left foot off the floor. Then jump to your left on the left foot, raising your right foot off the floor when you land. Repeat these movements continuously.

TRAINER'S TIP: Keep your chest up and use your arms to counterbalance.

BEGINNERS: Step out to the side rather than jump, but try to keep your trailing leg off the floor.

5. TUCK JUMPS

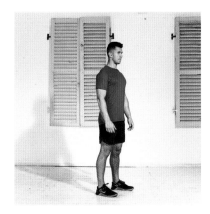 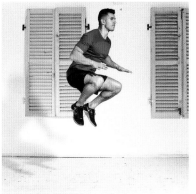 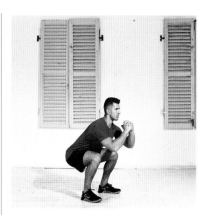

Stand with your feet shoulder-width apart. Jump your knees up as high as you can, then land. Repeat continuously.

TRAINER'S TIP: Keep your torso upright and your upper arms tucked into the sides of your body. Hold your hands out in front of you, with your lower arms parallel to the floor and palms facing down – try to tuck your knees up to your hands when you jump.

BEGINNERS: Swap the jumps for basic squats.

6. MOUNTAIN CLIMBERS

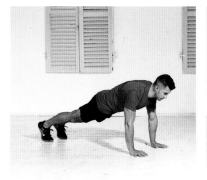 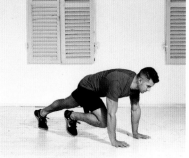 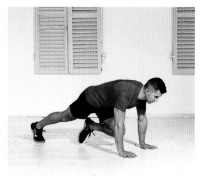

Get into plank position, with your feet hip-width apart. Take your right foot off the floor and crunch your right knee to your chest, then return to plank. Repeat, alternating legs.

TRAINER'S TIP: Keep your shoulders over your wrists to stop the body rocking forward. Try to pick up the pace so you are almost in a running motion.

BEGINNERS: Slow down the pace.

THE ONLY WORKOUT YOU WILL EVER REGRET IS THE ONE YOU DIDN'T DO, SO LET'S DRIVE THOSE KNEES INTO THAT CHEST AND SEE THIS THROUGH TO THE END.

7. SIT-UP PUNCHES

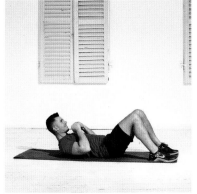 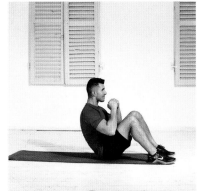 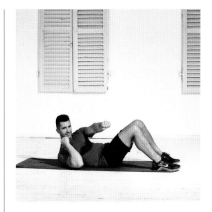

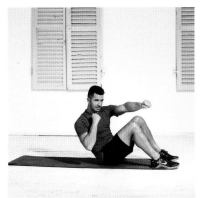

Lie on your back with your knees bent at a 90° angle and your feet flat on the floor. Engage your core and raise your head off the floor. Raise your arms into boxing position in front of your chest. From this starting position, crunch your back off the floor to bring your chest toward your knees, then cross jab with your right and left fists. Return to the starting position and repeat.

TRAINER'S TIP: Keep your feet flat on the floor as much as possible. When punching, cross your right fist over your left knee, and your left fist over your right knee.

BEGINNERS: Just crunch your shoulders up off the floor rather than your entire back.

8. TRICEP PUSH-UPS

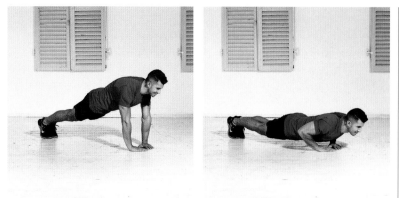 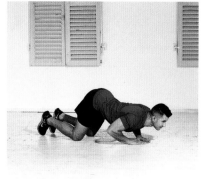

Get into plank position, with your feet together and your hands positioned close together, with thumbs touching. Lower your chest to the floor, then push up back to plank. Repeat.

TRAINER'S TIP: Always kiss your chest to the floor and look down.

BEGINNERS: Drop to your knees, but still try to kiss your chest to the floor.

9. PLANK PUNCHES

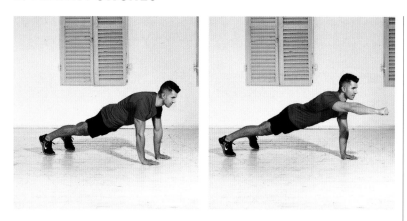 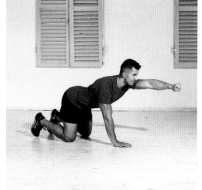

In a plank position, punch directly forward in front of your face with your right hand, then return to plank. Repeat, alternating arms.

TRAINER'S TIP: Keep your hips parallel to the floor and your feet shoulder-width apart.

BEGINNERS: Drop to your knees to perform this movement.

10. BURPEES

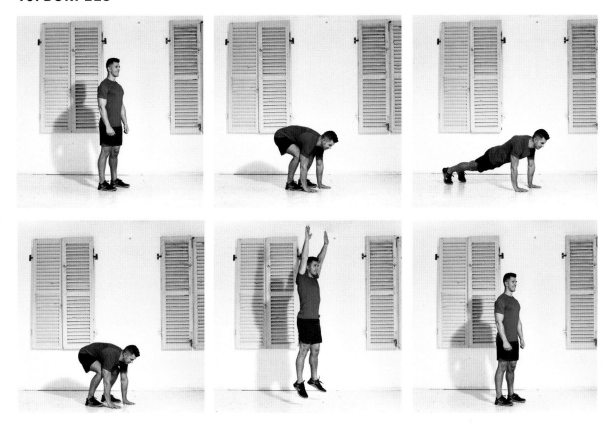

Stand with your feet hip-width apart. Bend down and place your hands on the floor in front of your feet, then jump your feet back into plank position. Now jump the feet back to your hands, then jump your body off the floor and raise your arms up in the air. Land back in standing position and repeat.

TRAINER'S TIP: To advance this move, lower your whole body to the floor, so your chest touches the ground, before explosively jumping up.

BEGINNERS: Step (rather than jump) your feet back to plank position, then back to your hands. Stand yourself up rather than jumping.

HALFWAY THERE. YOU'VE HEARD THE SAYING "REPETITION IS THE KEY TO SUCCESS", RIGHT? WELL, GUESS WHAT? RETURN TO THE FIRST MOVE BECAUSE WE ARE DOING 1—10 ALL OVER AGAIN. THEN TURN TO MY COOL-DOWN RECOVERY SEQUENCE ON PAGES 122—7.

WEEK TWO
DAY ONE/MONDAY
ARMS AND ABS

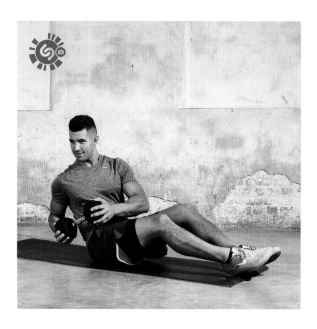

1. **WALKOUTS** (*see* page 47)

2. **PLANK T-ROTATIONS** (*see* page 48)

3. **ALTERNATING JACK KNIVES** (*see* page 49)

4. **PLANK SWIVELS** (*see* page 48)

5. **PLANK SHOULDER TAPS** (*see* page 47)

6. **DUMBBELL BICEP CURL TO SHOULDER PRESS** (*see* page 51)

7. **DUMBBELL OVERHEAD TRICEP EXTENSION** (*see* page 50)

8. **DUMBBELL BICEP CURLS** (*see* page 49)

9. **DUMBBELL TRICEP KICK-BACKS** (*see* page 51)

10. **DUMBBELL KNEELING SHOULDER PRESS** (*see* page 50)

11. **DUMBBELL BICEP CURL TO FOREHEAD** (*see* page 56)

12. **DUMBBELL PUSH PRESS** (*see* page 56)

13. **DUMBBELL ALTERNATING TRICEP KICK-BACKS** (*see* page 55)

14. **DUMBBELL ARNOLD PRESS** (*see* page 55)

15. **DUMBBELL CLOSE GRIP HAMMER CURLS** (*see* page 54)

16. **DUMBBELL PLANK PASSES** (*see* page 54)

17. **DUMBBELL SIT-UP REACHES** (*see* page 53)

18. **DUMBBELL V-SIT SHOULDER PRESS** (*see* page 53)

19. **DUMBBELL RAISED LEG TOE TOUCHES** (*see* page 52)

20. **DUMBBELL RUSSIAN TWISTS** (*see* page 52)

WEEK TWO
DAY TWO/TUESDAY
LEGS AND BUTT

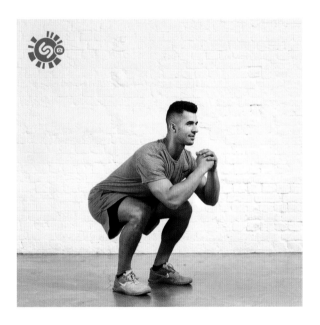

1. **CURTSEY LUNGE** (*see* page 61)
2. **TEMPO SQUATS 4-1** (*see* page 60)
3. **SIDE LUNGES** (*see* page 60)
4. **SQUATS** (*see* page 59)
5. **LUNGES** (*see* page 59)
6. **DUMBBELL CURTSEY LUNGE** (*see* page 63)
7. **DUMBBELL TEMPO SQUATS 4-1** (*see* page 63)
8. **DUMBBELL SIDE LUNGES** (*see* page 62)
9. **DUMBBELL SQUATS** (*see* page 62)
10. **DUMBBELL LUNGES** (*see* page 61)
11. **DUMBBELL KNEELING TO STANDING** (*see* page 69)
12. **DUMBBELL FRONT KICKS** (*see* page 68)
13. **DUMBBELL SWING SQUATS** (*see* page 68)
14. **DUMBBELL REVERSE LUNGES** (*see* page 67)
15. **DUMBBELL SUMO SQUATS** (*see* page 67)
16. **LUNGE JUMPS** (*see* page 66)
17. **DROP SQUATS** (*see* page 66)
18. **RIGHT LEG RUNNER'S LUNGE** (*see* page 65)
19. **LEFT LEG RUNNER'S LUNGE** (*see* page 65)
20. **SQUAT JUMPS** (*see* page 64)

WEEK TWO
DAY THREE/WEDNESDAY
CHEST, BACK AND CORE

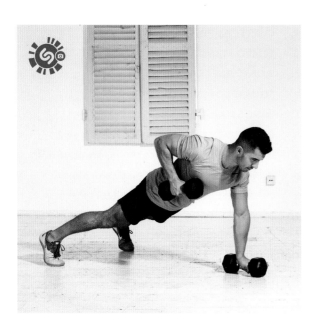

1. **PUSH UP TO REACH** (*see* page 73)
2. **PLANK** (*see* page 72)
3. **PLANK HIP TOUCH** (*see* page 72)
4. **SUPERMAN/SUPERWOMAN** (*see* page 71)
5. **T-ROTATION** (*see* page 71)
6. **DUMBBELL CHEST PRESS – PRONATED GRIP** (*see* page 73)
7. **DUMBBELL OVERHEAD PULLS** (*see* page 76)
8. **DUMBBELL CIRCULAR CHEST PRESS** (*see* page 75)
9. **DUMBBELL SEE-SAW PRESS – NEUTRAL GRIP** (*see* page 74)
10. **DUMBBELL CLOSE GRIP PRESS** (*see* page 74)
11. **RIGHT ELBOW TO LEFT KNEE CRUNCH** (*see* page 79)
12. **LEFT ELBOW TO RIGHT KNEE CRUNCH** (*see* page 79)
13. **RIGHT ARM SIDE PLANK DIPS** (*see* page 78)
14. **REVERSE PLANK HOLD** (*see* page 77)
15. **LEFT ARM SIDE PLANK DIPS** (*see* page 77)
16. **DUMBBELL DEADLIFT TO HIGH PULL** (*see* page 83)
17. **DUMBBELL RENEGADE ROWS** (*see* page 82)
18. **DUMBBELL BENT-OVER WIDE ROWS** (*see* page 81)
19. **DUMBBELL HIGH PULLS** (*see* page 81)
20. **DUMBBELL DEADLIFTS** (*see* page 80)

WEEK TWO
DAY FOUR/THURSDAY
ABS AND CORE

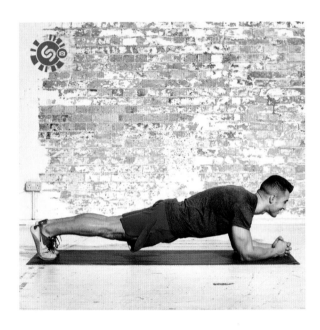

1. **PLANK SEE-SAW** (*see* page 90)

2. **RIGHT SIDE PLANK HOLD** (*see* page 90)

3. **ELBOW PLANK** (*see* page 89)

4. **LEFT SIDE PLANK HOLD** (*see* page 89)

5. **PLANK TUCKS** (*see* page 88)

6. **TWISTING MOUNTAIN CLIMBERS** (*see* page 88)

7. **PLANK JUMPING JACKS** (*see* page 87)

8. **STAR JUMPS** (*see* page 87)

9. **STANDING KNEE CRUNCH** (*see* page 85)

10. **HIGH KNEES** (*see* page 86)

NOW REPEAT THIS 10-MOVE WORKOUT

FULL BODY WITH WEIGHTS

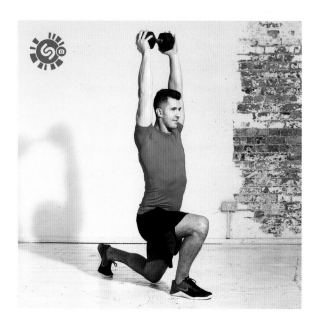

1. **PUSH-UPS** (*see* page 94)

2. **ELBOW PLANK** (*see* page 95)

3. **PIKE PUSH-UPS** (*see* page 95)

4. **WALKOUTS** (*see* page 93)

5. **PLANK** (*see* page 94)

6. **DUMBBELL LUNGE BICEP CURLS** (*see* page 99)

7. **DUMBBELL SHOULDER T-RAISES** (*see* page 99)

8. **DUMBBELL SQUAT PRESS** (*see* page 98)

9. **DUMBBELL SQUAT TRICEP EXTENSION** (*see* page 97)

10. **DUMBBELL SQUAT CURLS** (*see* page 96)

11. **WALKOUTS** (*see* page 106)

12. **PLANK** (*see* page 105)

13. **PUSH-UPS** (*see* page 105)

14. **ELBOW PLANK** (*see* page 104)

15. **PIKE PUSH-UPS** (*see* page 104)

16. **DUMBBELL WOOD CHOPS** (*see* page 103)

17. **DUMBBELL FROG SQUATS** (*see* page 103)

18. **DUMBBELL RIGHT LEG DEADLIFT TO CURL** (*see* page 102)

19. **DUMBBELL LEFT LEG DEADLIFT TO ROW** (*see* page 101)

20. **DUMBBELL OVERHEAD LUNGES** (*see* page 100)

WEEK TWO
DAY SIX/SATURDAY

FULL BODY, NO WEIGHTS

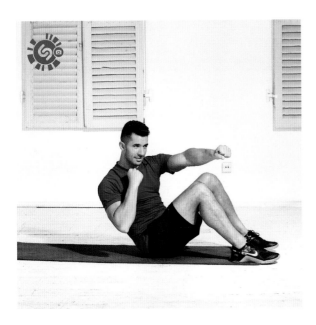

1. **TUCK JUMPS** (*see* page 111)
2. **LATERAL JUMPS** (*see* page 111)
3. **SQUAT PUNCHES** (*see* page 110)
4. **HIGH KNEE PUNCHES** (*see* page 109)
5. **QUICK FEET** (*see* page 109)
6. **BURPEES** (*see* page 115)
7. **PLANK PUNCHES** (*see* page 114)
8. **TRICEP PUSH-UPS** (*see* page 114)
9. **SIT-UP PUNCHES** (*see* page 113)
10. **MOUNTAIN CLIMBERS** (*see* page 112)

NOW REPEAT THIS 10-MOVE WORKOUT

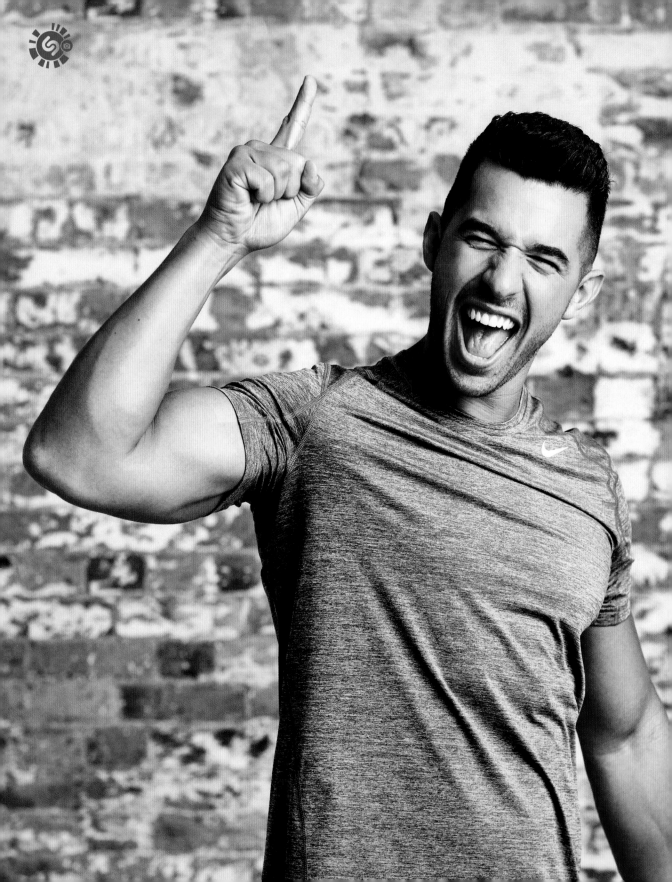

COOL DOWN AND RECOVERY

1. LIE FLAT – 30 SECONDS

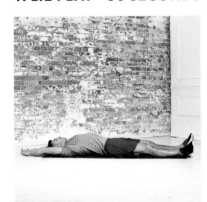

Lie flat on your back, with your arms and legs fully extended to make your body long.

TRAINER'S TIP: Use controlled breathing, inhaling through your nose and exhaling from your mouth, to lower the heart rate.

2. KNEE HUG – 30 SECONDS

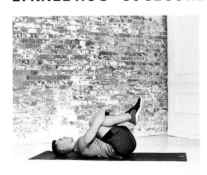

Still lying down, hug both your knees tight into your chest and gently rock from side to side or back and forth.

TRAINER'S TIP: Stay on your back when rocking – avoid rolling over onto your side – and breathe slowly.

3. FIGURE-OF-FOUR GLUTE STRETCH – 30 SECONDS

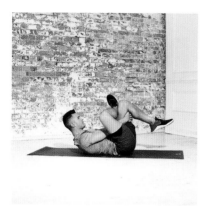

Still lying down, extend your legs upward. Drop your right ankle over your left knee to create a figure of four with your legs. Now, raise your shoulders off the floor, reach with both hands behind your left knee and pull it in toward your chest. Hold for 15 seconds, then repeat on the other side.

TRAINER'S TIP: Keep pulling your knee in toward your chest and see if you can push the bent knee of your uppermost leg away from you simultaneously, to progress the stretch in the glutes.

4. RIGHT LEG CIRCLES – 30 SECONDS

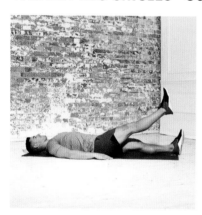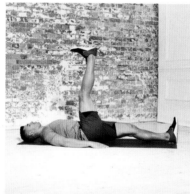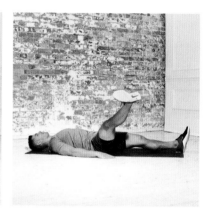

Lie flat on the floor with your arms by your sides, palms on the floor. Raise your right leg as high as you can. Keeping your right leg straight, move it out to the right from the hip, then down and round toward your left leg, then back up to the sky, moving the right leg in a big circle. Repeat in a continuous circular motion, making the circles as big as you can according to your flexibility.

TRAINER'S TIP: Keep the foot of the lifted leg flexed and the leg straight at all times.

5. LEFT LEG CIRCLES - 30 SECONDS

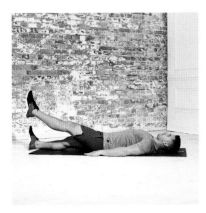 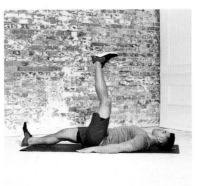 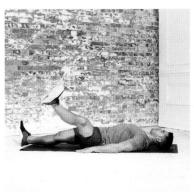

Follow the instructions for Right Leg Circles, but switch legs to make the circular motion with your left leg.

6. UP/DOWN DOG - 30 SECONDS

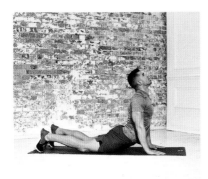 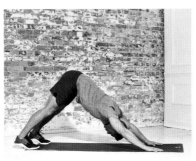

Lie down on your front, with your palms on the floor either side of your head. Extend your arms to raise your upper body off the floor and look up to the ceiling. Keep your hips on the floor in the up-dog position. Next, keeping your hands where they are, lower your head toward the floor and pike your hips up to the ceiling. Keep your legs straight and bring your head through your shoulders into the down-dog position. Repeat, moving fluidly between the two movements.

TRAINER'S TIP: Keep your breathing deep and slow and hold each position for a few seconds if you want to get deep into the stretch.

7. QUAD ROCKERS – 30 SECONDS

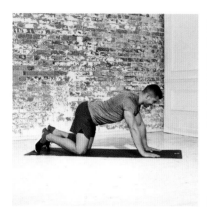 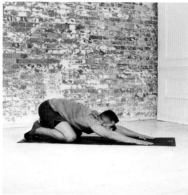

Kneel on all fours with your hands below your shoulders and your knees below your hips. Keeping your hands and knees in position, rock your bum back to your heels and stretch out your arms into child's pose, then return to all fours. Keep rocking between the two positions for 30 seconds.

TRAINER'S TIP: Stay dynamic by continuously moving through the movements. Keep your breathing controlled.

8. STANDING ROUNDED BACK – 10 SECONDS

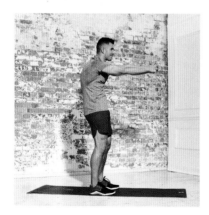

Stand with your feet shoulder-width apart. Interlink your fingers and reach out in front of you, rounding out your back. Hold for 10 seconds.

TRAINER'S TIP: Keep your hands level with your shoulders.

9. STANDING REACHES – 20 SECONDS

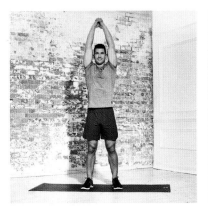 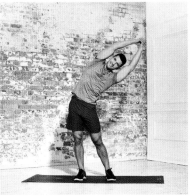 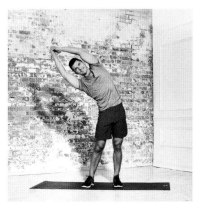

Stand with your feet shoulder-width apart. Reach your arms up to the ceiling and interlink your fingers. Now inhale and bend over to your left. Hold the stretch for 10 seconds, then return to centre. Inhale and repeat on the right.

TRAINER'S TIP: Allow your hips to move naturally and freely. Keep your body as long as possible.

10. STANDING SWEEPS TO PMA

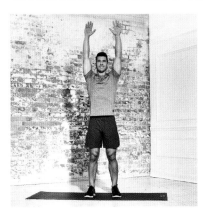 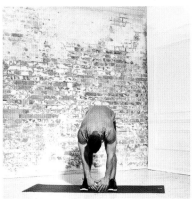 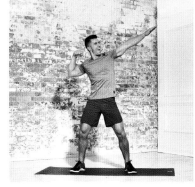

Standing tall, reach up to the ceiling with your hands. Now swing down, bending your body forward, and brush the floor with your fingers, then rise back to standing. Repeat this three times and, after the third rep, keep your body tall and reach up to the sky. Clench your fists and slowly visualize yourself pulling down your Positive Mental Attitude. Do my PMA pose if you feel like it!

TRAINER'S TIP: Try to keep your legs straight the whole time and, when you pull down that PMA, you had better mean it!

CHAPTER 5

THE RECIPES

Here's the part where you get to drool over lots of nice food pictures! You've got some breakfast, lunch and dinner options to see you through the week, plus a few snacks and a handful of cheat day recipes. Don't say I never treat you!

To recap:

- If you have not trained, make the standard recipe as it is. If you have worked out within the last 90 minutes, add on the pimp it up post-workout option to top up those carbs.
- If you are on a #MeatfreeMonday or just looking for a vegetarian recipe, all non-meat recipes, or recipes that provide alternative vegetation options, are labelled #MeatfreeMonday.
- If you are craving a takeaway, step away from the phone and flick though my recipes to find a healthier alternative. Just search for the #FaisalFakeaway tag.
- For those of you enjoying a #CheatDay, some of my favourite cheat-day recipes are included at the back of this recipe section. These are healthier versions of shop-bought treats because they're freshly made without the preservatives, but they still taste incredible. Just don't get excited by the word "healthier" – these are strictly cheat-day-only recipes.

Opposite: Turn my Prawn Taco Bowls with Zingy Slaw (see page 167) into a Mexican sharing feast the next time you have friends for dinner. Get stuck in and lick those fingers clean when you're done!

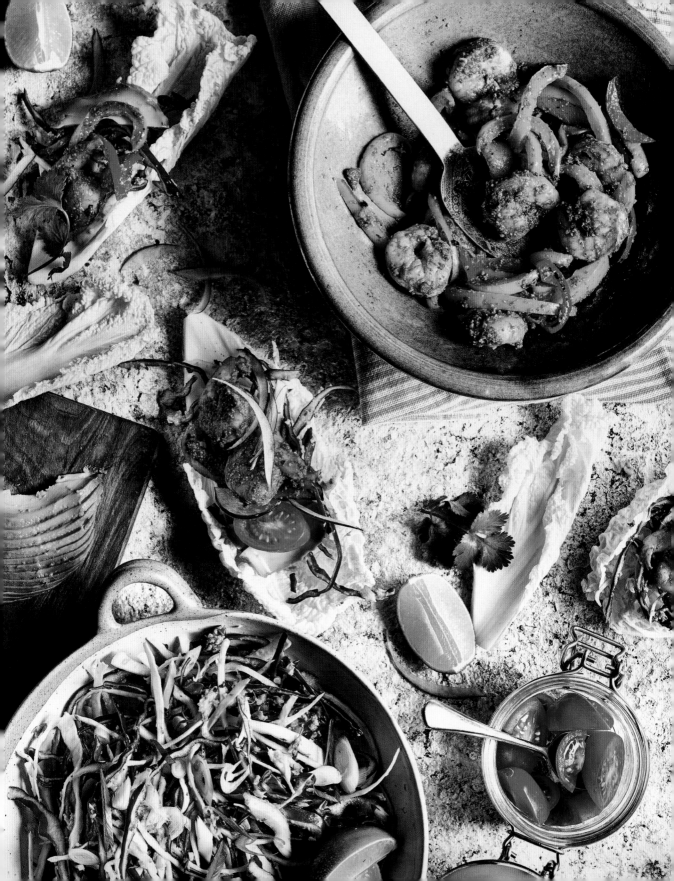

BREAKFAST

CHIA OVERNIGHT YOGURT
#MEATFREEMONDAY

SERVES 1

This is a super easy, roll-out-of-bed-and-eat-it breakfast for when you are having one of those mornings – Monday, you know what I'm talking about. There is nothing fancy about this, but it is high protein, gives a good dose of healthy fats and is so much better than the sugar-laden yogurts you so often find in shops. It is also a brilliant breakfast to eat post-workout and, if you make a few batches one night, you are good to go for two or three days.

Mix all of the ingredients in a bowl until thoroughly combined.

Refrigerate overnight and then eat for breakfast the following day.

200g (7oz) Greek yogurt
1½ tablespoons smooth peanut butter or almond butter
1 tablespoon chia seeds
2 tablespoons nut milk (almond milk works well)
1 teaspoon cacao powder
4 strawberries, sliced

PIMP IT UP POST-WORKOUT

Add 4 tablespoons of porridge oats and an extra 2 tablespoons of nut milk to the yogurt before refrigerating it and add half a sliced or mashed banana in the morning.

TIP:

Don't waste the other half of the banana you add post-workout. Freeze it for when you fancy a simple post-workout or cheat-day milkshake and blend it up with some almond milk.

FOUR-INGREDIENT PANCAKE STACK
#MEATFREEMONDAY

SERVES 2

Pancakes always feel like the ultimate indulgence, but they don't have to be made with flour and sugar to taste good. These contain just four ingredients, and are lovely just as they are, but I like to add a touch of sweetness with cinnamon and vanilla essence – and on cheat day I go all out and add chocolate chips, nut butter or blueberries before drowning them in maple syrup. Give it a go, you know you want to…

Put the cottage cheese, rolled oats, eggs and bicarbonate of soda into a blender. Add the cinnamon and vanilla, if using. Blend until the mixture is smooth. I don't blend for more than about 10 seconds so the batter retains some thickness.

This quantity of batter yields 6-12 pancakes, depending on the size you prefer. Whichever size you go for, you'll need to cook them in 2-3 batches. Put 1 teaspoon oil into a large nonstick frying pan over medium–low heat. Spoon the batter into the pan and use the back of the spoon to smooth the batter into neat circles. Ensure they are not too thick at the centres. I normally go for about 2 heaped tablespoons per pancake, which makes about 12, giving you 6 small pancakes per person.

Cook for about 1 minute, until bubbles begin to appear, then flip over and cook for a further minute or so until golden brown. Repeat with the remaining batter. Serve with the Greek yogurt and strawberries and decorate with sweet cinnamon, if using.

For the pancakes:
100g (3½oz) cottage cheese
100g (3½oz) rolled oats
  (the chunky variety)
4 eggs
1 teaspoon bicarbonate of soda
2–3 teaspoons coconut oil

Suggested add-ins (optional):
1 teaspoon ground sweet
  cinnamon, plus extra
  to decorate
½ teaspoon vanilla essence

Suggested toppings (optional):
2 tablespoons Greek yogurt
handful of strawberries

PIMP IT UP POST-WORKOUT

Substitute 2 tablespoons chocolate or vanilla protein powder for the vanilla essence and cinnamon. Stir a small handful of dark chocolate chips into the blended mix before cooking. Chop up a banana and mix it into 2 tablespoons Greek yogurt as a topping.

TIP:

For savoury pancakes, omit any sweet add-ins and add a bit of cheese, paprika and chives to the basic batter.

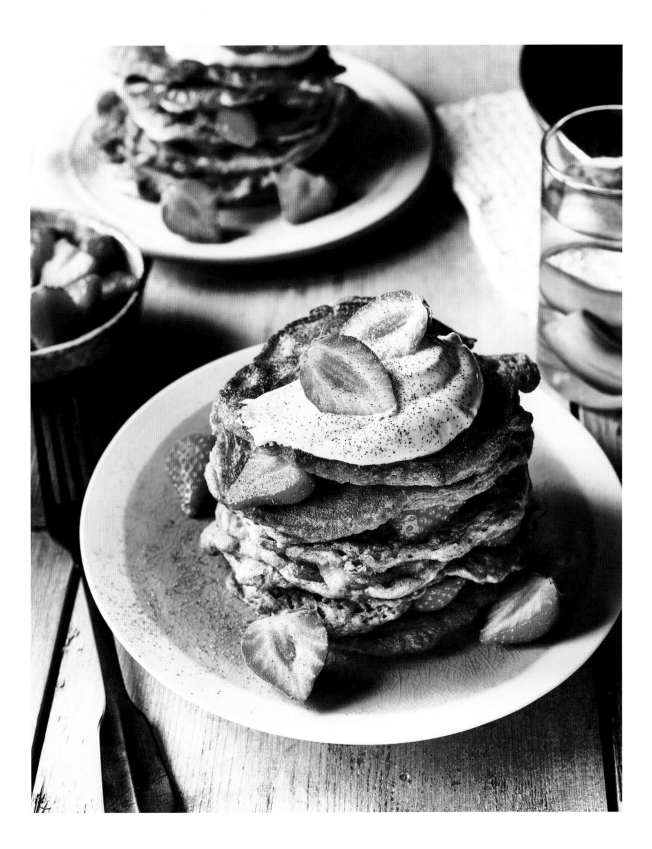

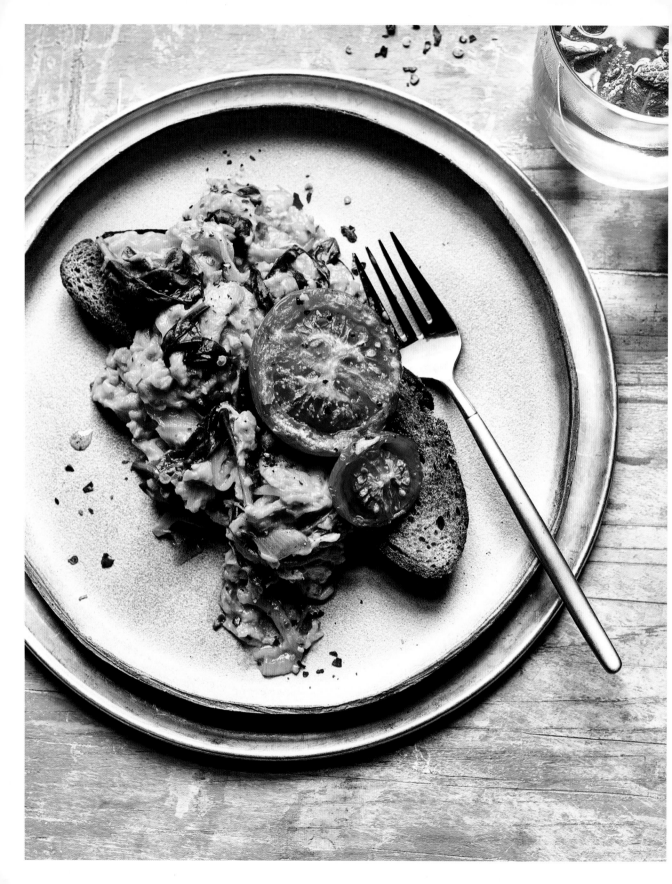

TURMERIC SCRAMBLED EGGS WITH ROASTED TOMATOES #MEATFREEMONDAY

SERVES 2

Hands up who is bored of normal scrambled eggs? This version contains turmeric, which has been used in India to treat inflammation for donkey's years, and has recently become a popular ingredient in the West as people catch on to its health benefits. This dish is a favourite of mine as a late breakfast after training, especially because it contains spinach, so I can have my Popeye moment.

To make the roasted tomatoes, preheat the oven to 200°C (400°F), Gas Mark 6.

Put all the ingredients for the tomatoes in a baking dish and mix together well so the tomatoes are nicely coated. Arrange the tomatoes in the dish, cut-sides up. Roast for about 15 minutes, until soft and juicy. (Alternatively, roast them for 45 minutes at 160°C (325°F), Gas Mark 3 if you prefer them slow-roasted.)

To make the eggs, melt the coconut oil in a frying pan over medium–low heat. Add the onion and garlic and cook for about 5 minutes, until softened, being careful not to burn them.

Meanwhile, put the grated turmeric into a bowl with the egg. Add the coconut milk and whisk together.

Once the onion is softened and becoming translucent, add the spinach and chilli flakes and cook for about 30 seconds until the leaves start to wilt. Pour in the egg mixture. Leave to cook around the edges slightly for about 20 seconds then, using a wooden spoon, pull the mixture in from the edges toward the centre of the pan and stir. Repeat until the eggs are almost cooked through. Take the eggs off the heat just before they are fully cooked, while still glistening and runny in places, as they continue to cook off the heat in the pan. Serve immediately, garnished with chilli flakes and with the roast tomatoes alongside.

For the eggs:
1 teaspoon coconut oil
½ white onion, finely sliced
1 garlic clove, crushed
2 teaspoons peeled and grated fresh turmeric (or use 1 teaspoon ground turmeric, but fresh is better here)
4 eggs
50ml (2fl oz) coconut milk
2 handfuls of spinach leaves
1 pinch of chilli flakes, plus extra to garnish

For the roasted tomatoes:
2 tomatoes, halved
drizzle of olive oil
pinch of salt
pinch of pepper
large pinch of garlic granules

PIMP IT UP POST-WORKOUT

Serve your eggs on a nice slice of toasted rye bread.

KICKING SCRAMBLED EGGS

Eggs are one of the few foods considered a "complete" protein, as they contain all the essential amino acids we need for everything, from fat burning and energy to stress relief and transporting nutrients around the body. Bottom line is, eggs are eggcellent (sorry). And they're great for breakfast as they help stave off those mid-morning cravings. This dish gives scrambled eggs a nice spicy twist. Serve it with Roasted Tomatoes (*see* page 135), adding ½ teaspoon dried thyme to the roasting mix, or my Smoky Baked Beans (*see* pages 140–1).

Heat 1 teaspoon of the oil in a frying pan over medium heat. Add the onion, jalapeño and turkey bacon and fry for about 5 minutes, until the onion is softened and translucent and the bacon is cooked through.

Meanwhile, whisk together the eggs, black pepper, coriander and the remaining oil in a bowl.

Add the tomatoes to the pan and cook for about 30 seconds. Pour in the egg mixture. Leave to cook around the edges slightly for about 20 seconds then, using a wooden spoon, pull the mixture in from the edges toward the centre of the pan and stir. Repeat until the eggs are almost cooked through. Take the eggs off the heat just before they are fully cooked, while still glistening and runny in places, as they continue to cook off the heat in the pan.

Transfer to serving plates. Garnish with the crumbled feta cheese and coriander and serve immediately.

- 2½ teaspoons olive oil
- ½ white onion, finely sliced
- 1 jalapeño chilli, deseeded and finely chopped
- 2 turkey bacon rashers, diced
- 4 eggs
- large pinch of ground black pepper
- 2 tablespoons chopped fresh coriander, plus a pinch extra to garnish
- 2 large plum tomatoes, deseeded and chopped
- a little crumbled feta cheese, to garnish

PIMP IT UP POST-WORKOUT

Add a slice of toasted rye bread.

BOILED EGG AND DIPPY SOLDIERS

SERVES 2

Who didn't love dipping soldiers into runny eggs as a kid? As with a lot of things in life, I've never grown out of it. This recipe uses crispy turkey bacon-wrapped asparagus as the dippy soldiers, because I have to pretend to be an adult now. The bacon gives an extra hit of protein, while the asparagus, a superhero vegetable, brings good levels of vitamin C to the party and promotes healthy gut bacteria.

Preheat your grill on a high setting.

Wrap 1 turkey bacon rasher around the length of 1 asparagus spear, pulling it taut as you go to wrap the spear tightly. Try not to overlap the bacon so it cooks evenly. Repeat with the remaining turkey bacon rashers and 3 of the remaining asparagus spears.

Lay the bacon-wrapped asparagus spears in a grill pan with the bacon ends tucked under so they don't unravel. Grill for 10–15 minutes, turning half way through, until the bacon becomes crispy, adding the unwrapped spears for the final 6–7 minutes.

Meanwhile, bring a saucepan of water to the boil, then reduce the heat to produce a quick simmer. Carefully drop in the eggs and simmer for as long as you like, depending on how you like your eggs cooked. I aim for 6 minutes for a runny soft-boiled egg if I have 4 eggs in the pan. Remove the eggs with a slotted spoon and transfer to eggcups.

Serve 2 eggs, 2 bacon-wrapped asparagus spears and 1 plain asparagus spear per person.

4 streaky turkey bacon rashers
6 asparagus spears, woody ends snapped off
4 eggs

PIMP IT UP POST-WORKOUT

Toast a slice of rye bread per person and let it get involved with the dippy soldier crew.

#MEATFREEMONDAY

Lose the turkey bacon if you are vegetarian or on a Meatfree Monday.

TIP:

When you remove the boiled eggs from the water, pop in some more to boil, to prepare some filling snacks for the week. Once cooked, put them into cold water to cool, then refrigerate. I keep enough for 3 or 4 days so, if there's no time for breakfast, I can grab a couple of eggs – far better than a sugary cereal bar.

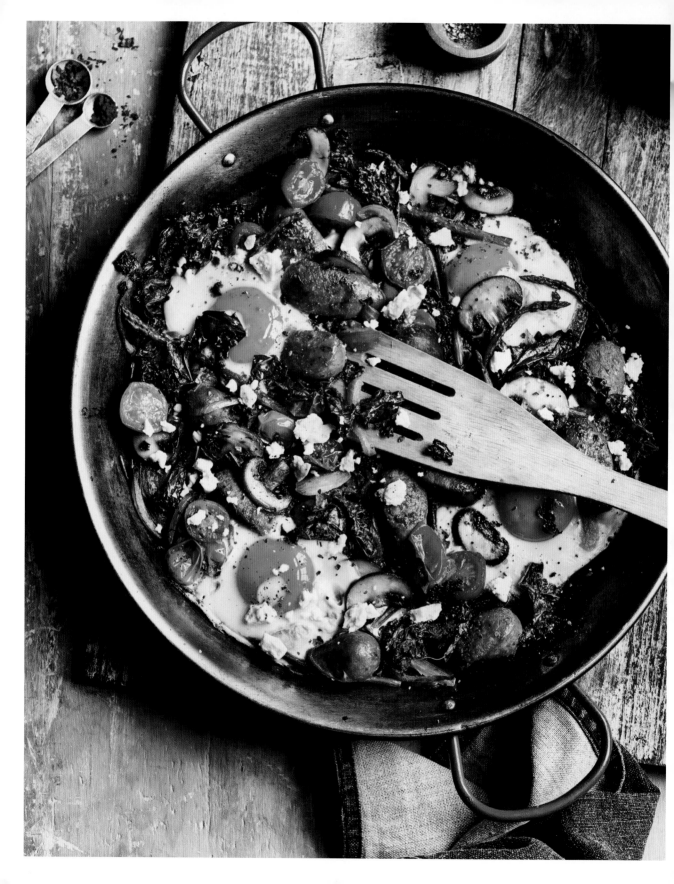

KITCHEN-SINK ONE-PAN BREAKFAST

We call this a kitchen-sink breakfast at home because we throw in everything but the kitchen sink. (And using just one pan means less washing up!) Play around and throw in whatever breakfast ingredients you fancy – bacon, mushrooms, red pepper, salmon, chorizo, you name it. If you plan to eat the pimped-up version after a morning workout, cook your sausages and sweet potato the night before so you can knock it up quickly after training.

Heat the oil in a frying pan over medium heat. Fry the sausages until golden and cooked through, about 5 minutes, depending on the size of your sausages. Drain off any excess fat, then return the pan with the sausages to the heat.

Add the asparagus and red onion and fry for a couple of minutes, stirring to prevent burning, until the onion begins to soften. Add the kale, tomatoes and all the herbs and spices and cook for a further minute, stirring now and then.

Make 4 little wells in the mixture toward the outside of the pan and crack an egg into each well. The eggs will take slightly longer than normal to cook because the pan is filled, but the whites should be cooked in about 4 minutes. Remove from the heat when the eggs are done to your liking.

Place the pan on a heatproof plate and serve your breakfast straight from the pan, crumbling over some feta before you tuck in.

1 teaspoon coconut oil

4 chicken sausages, cut into thirds

8 fine asparagus spears, woody ends snapped off

½ red onion, finely sliced

2 handfuls of kale, destalked and roughly chopped

8 cherry or baby plum tomatoes, halved

1 teaspoon garlic granules

1 teaspoon dried parsley

1 teaspoon paprika

½ teaspoon smoked paprika

pinch of ground black pepper

4 eggs

a little crumbled feta cheese, to garnish

PIMP IT UP POST-WORKOUT

Peel and thinly slice a small sweet potato and add it to the pan after draining the excess fat from the sausages. Fry for 5–7 minutes, stirring occasionally, until the sweet potato is tender, then continue with the remaining steps.

#MEATFREEMONDAY

Switch the sausages for Smoky Baked Beans (see pages 140–1) if you are vegetarian or enjoying a Meatfree Monday.

TIP:

I love crispy kale, where it is on the cusp of burning. It gives it a nice nutty flavour. Add your kale a bit earlier if you want it extra crispy around the edges.

POACHED EGG WITH SMOKY BAKED BEANS AND BUBBLE AND SQUEAK PATTIES #MEATFREEMONDAY

SERVES 4

Beans, beans, they're good for your heart, the more you eat, the more you... smile! Because these are so good! Shop-bought baked beans are often laden with hidden sugars, so avoid that trap and make your own. I serve them with poached eggs (which I have finally mastered after three decades, thanks to a great tip from Jamie Oliver) and some crispy veggie patties, which you can use to mop up all that runny yolk goodness.

First, prepare the patties. Bring a saucepan of water to a boil. Add the broccoli florets and boil for about 5 minutes, until the stems are soft. Drain thoroughly, then transfer to a bowl and mash well with a fork or potato masher.

Put the grated shallots and cheese into a large bowl. Add the mashed broccoli and the remaining ingredients, excluding the oil, and mix well. If the mixture looks too wet, add more ground almond. Set aside in the refrigerator until ready to cook the patties.

Now prepare the eggs for poaching. If you already poach a great egg, do it your way, but this method is ace. Take 4 ramekins, teacups or small bowls and rub the insides with a little olive oil using your fingers or kitchen paper. Now line each ramekin with a double layer of clingfilm, ensuring the clingfilm is at least double the size of the ramekin – aim for about 15-20 x 15-20cm (6-8 x 6-8 inches). Push the clingfilm down so that it tightly lines the ramekin, then rub olive oil around the areas of clingfilm inside the containers. Crack an egg into each ramekin, being careful not to break the yolks.

Working on 1 ramekin at a time, gather up the clingfilm so it forms a little bag. Gently push the yolk down into the egg white. Seal the bag by tying a knot in the clingfilm as close to the egg as possible. Set aside until ready to poach the eggs.

Bring a medium-large saucepan of water to the boil, then reduce the heat to produce a simmer.

Meanwhile, make the baked beans. Heat the oil in a frying pan over medium heat. Add the onion and garlic and cook for 2-3 minutes until softened. Stir in the smoked paprika, paprika, thyme and tomato purée and cook for 2 minutes.

For the eggs:
olive oil, for greasing
4 eggs

For the patties:
½ head of broccoli, broken into florets
2 shallots or ½ white onion, coarsely grated
2 thumb-sized pieces of Cheddar cheese, coarsely grated
1 egg, whisked
1 small handful of chopped spinach
3 tablespoons ground almonds, plus extra as required
1 teaspoon paprika
½ teaspoon garlic granules
¼ teaspoon ground black pepper
pinch of salt
1 teaspoon coconut oil

For the smoky baked beans:
1 tablespoon olive oil
½ red onion, finely diced
2 garlic cloves, crushed

Add the beans, passata, soy sauce and sriracha sauce, if using, and simmer for 5-7 minutes, until the sauce starts to thicken. Add the black pepper, then taste your sauce – stir in the maple syrup and some salt if you think it needs them.

While the beans are cooking, poach the eggs and cook the patties. Carefully place the egg pouches into the simmering water and poach for 5-7 minutes, until the whites are cooked. Pull the pouches out of the water, undo the clingfilm and serve immediately.

To cook the patties, heat the coconut oil in a frying pan over medium heat. When hot, divide your mixture into 4 portions and shape each into a patty. Cook for 3-4 minutes on each side, until golden. Flatten the patties slightly with a spatula when you flip them. The mixture may be a little loose to begin with, but will bind better as the egg cooks and the patties form a golden crust on the outside.

½ teaspoon smoked paprika
½ teaspoon paprika
½ teaspoon dried thyme
1 tablespoon tomato purée
400g (14oz) can cannellini
    beans, rinsed and drained
100g (3½oz) passata
1 tablespoon soy sauce
1 teaspoon sriracha sauce
    (optional)
large pinch of ground black
    pepper
½ tablespoon maple syrup,
    if needed
sea salt, to taste, if needed

TIP:

Make extra beans and refrigerate them for up to 2 days. They are even tastier the next day. Make this breakfast again, or add them to the pan when you cook my Kitchen-sink One-pan Breakfast (see page 139).

CHEESY SALMON, BROCCOLI AND DILL FRITTATA

SERVES 2-4

Frittatas must be up there as one of the easiest things to make. You can add whatever you want to the mix, so it never gets boring. This low-carb frittata is a good option if you have not got your training in before your breakfast. The salmon is a great source of high-quality protein and is bursting with omega 3, selenium and B vitamins. This dish offers a tasty way to pack in all that goodness, and the best part is that it is stupidly simple to make.

Bring a saucepan of water to the boil. Add the asparagus and broccoli, reduce the heat and simmer for 2 minutes to parboil. Drain and set aside.

Heat the olive oil in a large frying pan over medium heat. Add the salmon and fry for about 4 minutes, until cooked and flaking.

Meanwhile, mix half the grated cheese into the whisked eggs in a bowl.

When the salmon is ready, add the frozen peas, tomatoes, broccoli and asparagus to the pan. Ensure everything is well mixed and evenly spread out. Now add the eggs, herbs and garlic in quick succession and make sure the eggs are evenly spread, then sprinkle over the remaining Cheddar and a good pinch of black pepper.

Preheat the grill on a high setting.

Cook for about 2 minutes over medium heat, until the frittata is set on the base and sides. Transfer the pan to the grill and cook for 3-4 minutes or until the frittata is set.

Leave the frittata in the pan for a couple of minutes, then slide it out onto a plate and cut it into quarters. Enjoy warm for breakfast, garnished with dill fronds, or leave to cool, then refrigerate to enjoy cold over the next couple of days.

PIMP IT UP POST-WORKOUT

Cook my Sweet Potato, Red Pepper and Sausage Frittata instead (see page 144).

8 asparagus spears, woody ends snapped off, cut into thirds
½ head of broccoli, cut into bite-sized pieces
drizzle of olive oil
2 salmon fillets, about 130g (4½oz) each, cut into bite-sized pieces
50g (1¾oz) Cheddar cheese, grated
6 eggs, whisked
handful of frozen peas
6 cherry tomatoes, halved
1 tablespoon finely chopped dill, plus extra to garnish
2 tablespoons finely chopped chives
½ teaspoon garlic powder
pinch of ground black pepper

TIP:

Use the mixture to make muffin frittatas, an easily transportable breakfast or snack that you can eat with no mess. Preheat the oven to 190°C (375°F), Gas Mark 5. Lightly grease a 12-hole muffin tin with oil (you may need a second tin, depending on the size of your eggs). Leave out the tomatoes and chop the fish and vegetables into smaller pieces. Mix these in a bowl with the eggs, cheese and herbs. Spoon the mixture into the prepared tin and bake for about 20 minutes, until the tops are firm and set.

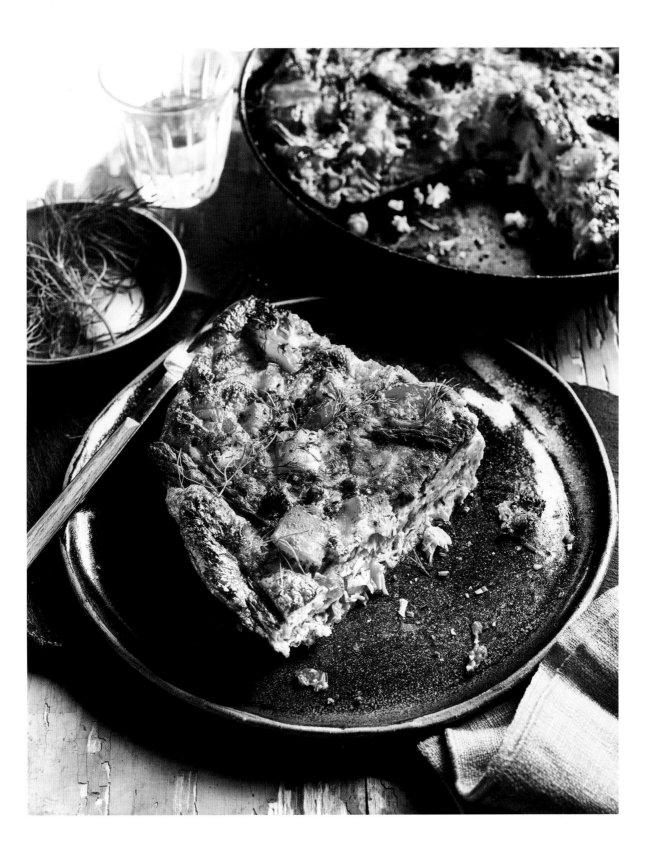

POST-WORKOUT SWEET POTATO, RED PEPPER AND SAUSAGE FRITTATA

SERVES 2-4

This one is a bit of an exception to the other recipes in this book, because the post-workout version is presented upfront, but that's because this is how I mostly make it. The sweet potato, red peppers and tomatoes make for an almost sweet frittata. It's a hearty breakfast to enjoy after a training session and I make it a lot because it's easy to cook and transport – great for a post-training lunch at the gym. But if you haven't worked out before breakfast, substitute two handfuls of spinach and a handful of frozen peas for the sweet potato.

Fry the sausages in a large, nonstick frying pan over medium heat for about 5 minutes, until browned. Drain off any excess fat, then add the sweet potato and fry together for another 5 minutes, stirring occasionally, until the sweet potato begins to soften.

Add the red peppers to the pan and cook for about 3-4 minutes, until the potatoes and peppers are tender. Mix in the tomatoes and garlic powder, add the whisked eggs, then sprinkle over half the crumbled feta, the dill, parsley and chilli flakes.

Preheat the grill on a high setting.

Cook for about 2 minutes, until the frittata is set on the base and sides. Crumble over the remaining feta, transfer to the grill and cook for 3-4 minutes or until the frittata is set.

Leave the frittata in the pan for a couple of minutes, then slide it out onto a plate and cut it into quarters. Enjoy warm for breakfast, or leave to cool, then refrigerate to enjoy cold over the next couple of days.

4 chicken sausages, cut into thirds
1 sweet potato, peeled and thinly sliced
2 red peppers, thinly sliced
2 tomatoes, quartered
1 teaspoon garlic powder
6 eggs, whisked
100g (3½oz) feta cheese, crumbled
1 tablespoon finely chopped dill
1 teaspoon dried parsley
pinch of chilli flakes
salt and pepper, to taste

MEXICAN HUEVOS RANCHEROS
#MEATFREEMONDAY

Thank you, Mexico, for this dish! It is smoky, spicy, fresh and creamy, all at once. I ate it almost every morning when I was there, but would have it for breakfast, lunch or dinner any time! I love it because it's a nice pan-on-the-table, dig-in-and-share type of meal. It also cooks up in no time if you batch cook the tomato sauce and freeze it, ready for whenever you fancy this meal. Also, it's a great dish for "cook-once, eat-twice" treatment – I happily eat this cold the next day and think the flavours are sometimes even better.

Heat the oil in a large frying pan over medium heat. Add the onion, garlic and pepper and cook for about 5 minutes, until soft. Add the jalapeño, paprika, ground coriander and chilli flakes and stir together for approximately 30 seconds.

Add the chopped tomatoes, bay leaves, smoked paprika and half the measured water to the pan, stir well, then reduce the heat to simmer for 10-15 minutes, until the sauce has thickened and reduced. Taste and season with the salt, then mix in the remaining water. Cook for 1 minute.

Remove the bay leaves. Using the back of a spoon, make 4 little wells in the sauce, then crack 1 egg into each well. Try to crack them in as quickly as possible so they cook at the same time. Cover the pan with a lid and cook for 4–6 minutes, until the egg whites are set but the yolks remain runny.

While the eggs are cooking, prepare the avocado garnish. Put the avocado into a bowl with the lime juice and mash them together with a fork. Set aside.

Place the pan on a heatproof plate on the table and serve straight from the pan. Top with sliced spring onion, chopped coriander, a little crumbling of feta and the avocado and lime mixture.

```
1 teaspoon olive oil
½ white onion, diced
2 garlic cloves, crushed
1 red pepper, diced
1 jalapeño chilli, deseeded
   and finely diced
1 teaspoon paprika
1 teaspoon ground coriander
½ teaspoon chilli flakes
400g (14oz) can chopped tomatoes
3 bay leaves
1 teaspoon smoked paprika
100ml (3½fl oz) water
pinch of sea salt
4 eggs

To garnish:
1 avocado
juice of ½ lime
2 spring onions, sliced
handful of fresh coriander,
   chopped
a little crumbled feta cheese
```

PIMP IT UP POST-WORKOUT

Warm 1 wholemeal tortilla per person to serve with this dish, or make up some Freakin' Fast Flatbreads (*see* page 182 – omit the garlic and coriander). Use your tortilla to make a Mexican breakfast wrap or to mop up the juices.

TIP:

This sauce also works well alongside my Baba's Beef Kofte (*see* page 156).

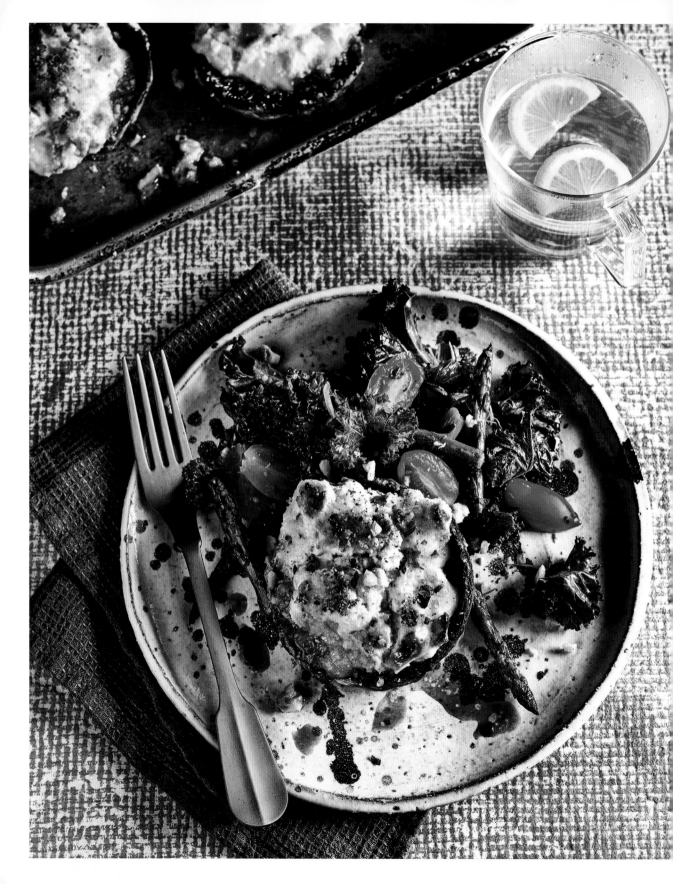

BLUE CHEESE-STUFFED MUSHROOMS WITH KALE MASH-UP #MEATFREEMONDAY

SERVES 2

These giant, cheesy stuffed mushrooms contain quark, a dairy product that's like a cross between Greek yogurt and cottage cheese. It is popular in Scandinavia, where they have cottoned on to its high protein content. You'll find it in most supermarkets. I add it to lots of recipes now because I'm a man who loves his protein gains! It's great in this moreish mushroom dish. With a big pile of greens, it'll give your day a great start.

Preheat the oven to 200°C (400°F), Gas Mark 6.

Lay the mushrooms on a baking tray with the gills facing up.

Mix the quark, blue cheese, walnuts and chilli flakes in a bowl and spoon the mixture into the mushrooms. Top with a generous layer of the ground almonds. Bake for 10 minutes, until the mushrooms have softened.

Meanwhile, preheat the grill on a high setting.

Transfer the baking tray to the grill and cook for 5–8 minutes, until the tops of the mushrooms are golden. If there are any juices in the bottom of the tray, pour them into a cup and set aside until ready to serve.

To make the kale, melt the coconut oil in a frying pan over medium heat. Add the asparagus and fry for about 1½ minutes, until slightly softened. Now add the kale, chilli flakes and garlic granules. Cook for another 1½ minutes, until the kale starts to wilt, shrink and soften.

Stir in the tomatoes and, after 30 seconds, the lemon juice, along with any reserved mushroom juices. Serve the kale alongside the mushrooms.

For the mushrooms:
2 large flat mushrooms (use 4 if you can't find the really big ones), stems removed
4 tablespoons quark cheese
35g (1¼oz) blue cheese, crumbled
25g (1oz) chopped walnuts
pinch of dried chilli flakes
2—2½ tablespoons ground almonds

For the kale:
½ teaspoon coconut oil
10 asparagus spears, woody ends snapped off, cut into thirds
3 handfuls of torn kale leaves, destalked
pinch of dried chilli flakes
½ teaspoon garlic granules
10 baby plum tomatoes, halved
2 tablespoons lemon juice

PIMP IT UP POST-WORKOUT

At the risk of sounding terribly boring, I quite like this with a slice of rye bread. Alternatively, finely slice a sweet potato and fry it in a little coconut oil for 6–8 minutes, then add the asparagus and follow the method above.

TIP:

Mushrooms are quite watery and I like to collect any excess juices when I cook them to use as seasoning, as I would soy sauce, in whatever else I'm cooking. Give it a go.

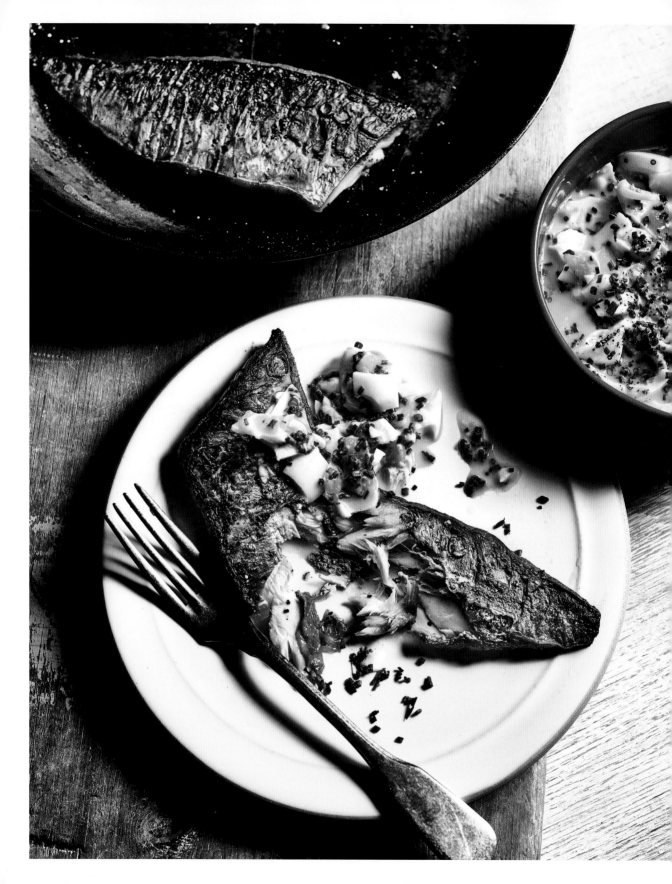

CAPE CLEAR MACKEREL AND GUGGIE EGG

SERVES 2

I have been visiting family in Cape Clear, a tiny island off the coast of Baltimore in Ireland, since I was a child. They do breakfast there like nowhere else. Freshly caught mackerel is a speciality, brought straight in from the sea to the cast iron cooker. I love it served with a guggie egg (an egg made in a cup).

To cook the eggs, bring a saucepan of water to the boil, then reduce the heat to produce a quick simmer. Carefully lower in the eggs and simmer for 6 minutes, depending on the size of the eggs (you want a nice runny yolk).

Meanwhile, cook the fish. Heat the oil in a frying pan over medium heat. Once the pan is hot add the fillets, skin-sides down, and fry for about 4 minutes until the skin is crispy. Sprinkle each fillet with a pinch of pepper, then flip over and cook for another 2 minutes, or until cooked through, adding the lemon juice in the final 15 seconds of cooking.

Once the cooking time for the eggs has elapsed, transfer to a bowl of cold water to halt the cooking process, then, as soon as they are cool enough to handle (so they remain warm), remove the shells.

Put the butter, vinegar, 1 tablespoon of the chives, the pepper and the eggs into a large cup or bowl. Use a knife to cut and mash up the egg a little bit, then stir everything together well. You should have a wet chopped egg mixture.

Serve the mackerel with the egg alongside, garnished with the remaining chives.

For the eggs:
4 eggs
1 teaspoon butter
1 teaspoon malt vinegar
1½ tablespoons finely chopped chives
large pinch of ground black pepper

For the fish:
1 teaspoon olive oil
2 skin-on mackerel fillets, about 90g (3¼oz) each
2 pinches of ground black pepper
2 tablespoons lemon juice

PIMP IT UP POST-WORKOUT

Add a lovely slice of toasted rye bread or some wholemeal toast and enjoy.

TIP:

If you ever fancy a high-protein snack, 1 guggie egg is perfect. Just adjust the quantities of the ingredients accordingly.

LUNCH

GARLIC-AND-CHILLI PRAWNS, TAPAS-STYLE

SERVES 2–3

If you're feeling super lazy but want a big bowlful of taste, packed with protein and healthy fats, look no further. This dish is ready in minutes and is perfect for enjoying in the garden with a good book and music… or sharing on Instagram, if you're anything like me! Make extra and enjoy it for lunch the next day, or eat the whole lot in one go if, again, you're anything like me!

Put the spinach and avocado into a large serving bowl and set aside.

Heat 1 teaspoon butter and the oil in a frying pan over medium heat. Add the garlic and prawns. Fry for about 1 minute, until the garlic begins to brown.

Stir in 2 tablespoons of the parsley and half the chilli and fry for another minute, then pour in half the lemon juice. Mix well, ensure the prawns are fully heated through, then remove them from the pan and transfer to the bowl with the spinach and avocado, leaving as much of the juice in the pan as possible.

Return the pan to the heat, add the remaining butter, lemon and chilli and the pepper and cook for about 45 seconds, until the butter begins to brown slightly. Drizzle the sauce around the prawns, onto the spinach leaves. Top with the remaining parsley and dig in!

4 large handfuls of spinach
1 avocado, diced
1 tablespoon plus 1 teaspoon butter
1 teaspoon olive oil
2 garlic cloves, crushed
300g (10½oz) cooked, peeled and deveined king prawns
3 tablespoons finely chopped flat leaf parsley
1 red chilli, deseeded and finely chopped
4 tablespoons lemon juice
large pinch of ground black pepper

PIMP IT UP POST-WORKOUT

Those juices were made for a chunk of wholemeal bread.

TIP:

Try garnishing the dish with a pinch of smoked paprika along with the parsley for added warmth and a Spanish touch.

NOT-MAMA'S JERK CHICKEN WITH MANGO AND BLACK BEAN SALSA #FAISALFAKEAWAY

SERVES 4

When I'm at Notting Hill Carnival there's only one jerk chicken stall I make my way to. I can never replicate the magic of Mama's jerk chicken, because her jerk seasoning is a secret family recipe, but I've fallen love with the dish, so here is my homage to it.

To prepare the rub for the chicken, put the chilli, ginger, spring onion and thyme into a food processor and pulse until finely chopped. Add the remaining ingredients, excluding the chicken and lime quarters, and pulse a few times until well mixed. The mixture should be quite stiff, not runny.

Score your chicken thighs or stab them a few times so the rub can penetrate the flesh. Put them into a large bowl, add the rub mixture and massage it into every nook and cranny of the meat. Transfer the chicken to a plastic storage container or freezer bag and seal. Leave in the refrigerator to marinate for a minimum of 1 hour or, if possible, overnight or throughout the day.

Preheat the oven to 220°C (425°F), Gas Mark 7. Put the chicken into a deep baking tray and roast in the centre of the oven for about 30 minutes, until golden and cooked through (the juices should run clear when the meat is pierced with a knife). Increase the oven temperature to 240°C (475°F), Gas Mark 9 and roast the chicken for a further 5 minutes, until the skin is crispy.

Meanwhile, make the mango black bean salsa. Mix all the ingredients together in a bowl and it's done!

Place the baking tray with the chicken on a heatproof plate on the table and serve straight from the pan. Garnish with the quartered limes and serve with the salsa.

PIMP IT UP POST-WORKOUT

Boil 50g (1¾oz) brown rice per person and add it to the salad or serve on the side.

#MEATFREEMONDAY

For a vegetarian option, substitute 4 x 100g (3½oz) tofu steaks for the chicken. Use 1 quartered red onion, 1 chopped red pepper, 1 chopped yellow pepper, 1 chopped aubergine and florets from ½ head of cauliflower. Follow the same process, rubbing the spice mixture into the vegetables and tofu, and roast at 200°C (400°F), Gas Mark 6 for 20–30 minutes.

1–2 Scotch bonnet chillies, deseeded

½ thumb-sized piece of fresh root ginger, peeled and finely chopped

6 spring onions, cut roughly into thirds

2 tablespoons thyme leaves or 1 tablespoon dried thyme

2 garlic cloves

1 tablespoon ground allspice

½ teaspoon ground cinnamon

½ teaspoon ground nutmeg

2 tablespoons soy sauce

1½ tablespoons maple syrup

juice of 1 lime

pinch of ground black pepper

glug of olive oil

8 skin-on and bone-in chicken thighs

2 limes, quartered, to garnish

For the black bean salsa:

400g (14oz) can black beans, rinsed and drained

1 red pepper, finely chopped

½ red onion, finely chopped

1 avocado, cut into small dice

250g (9oz) mango, peeled and chopped into bite-sized pieces (or buy a ready prepared packet)

juice of 1 lime

3 tablespoons freshly squeezed orange juice

2 tablespoons chopped fresh coriander

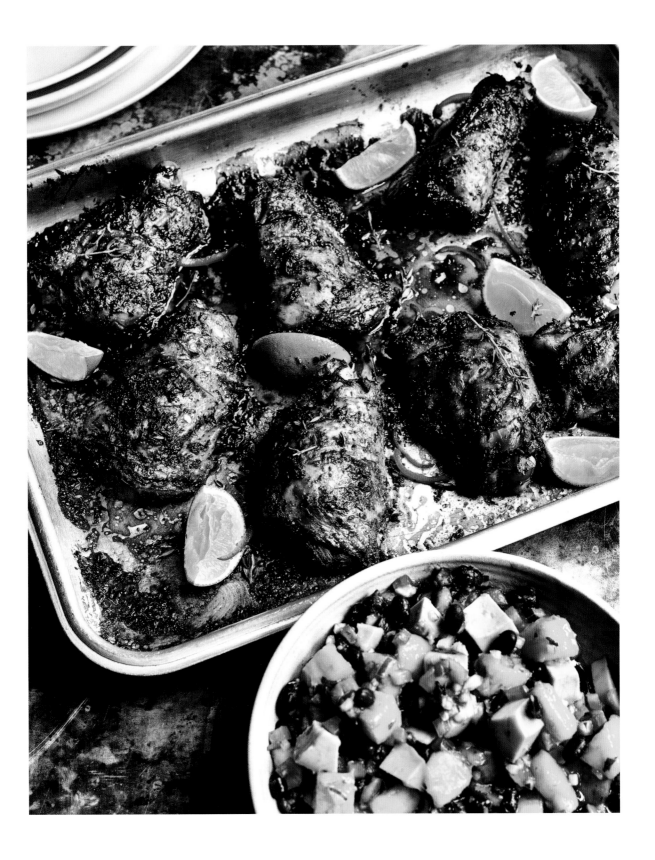

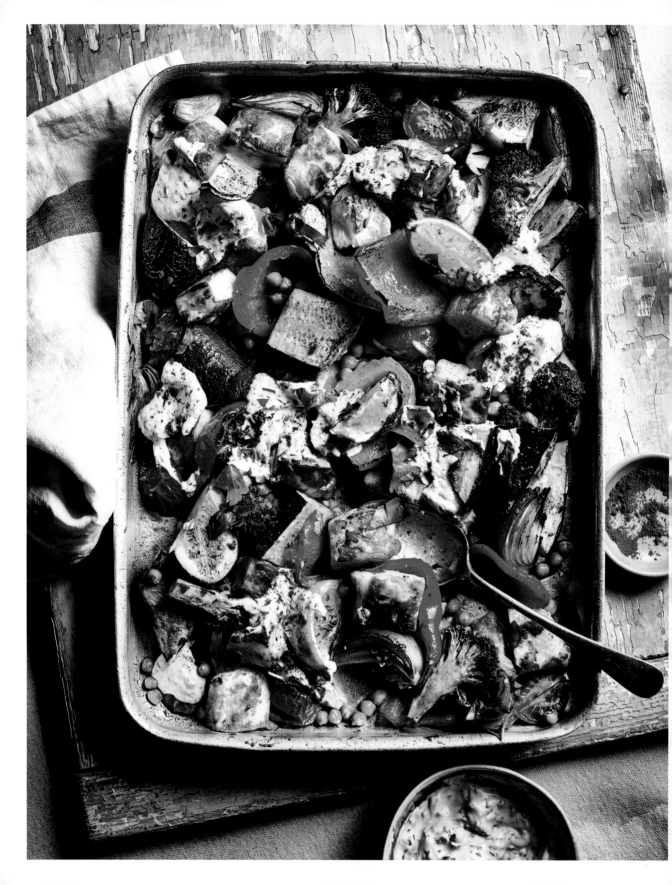

SMOKY HARISSA HALLOUMI
AND VEGETABLE TRAY BAKE
WITH PARSLEY YOGURT DRESSING
#MEATFREEMONDAY

SERVES 4

Tray bakes that you can shove into the oven to cook while you train are going to become your friend. This vegetarian dish combines salty halloumi with the smoky tones of harissa for a Moroccan-inspired dish that you can happily share with friends, or devour the leftovers the next day.

Preheat the oven to 190°C (375°F), Gas Mark 5.

Put the peppers, courgette, broccoli, onion and garlic cloves into a large, deep baking tray. Add the harissa, lemon juice and olive oil and give everything a good mix with your hands so all the vegetables are evenly coated. Add the chickpeas and lemon quarters to the tray. Bake for 30 minutes, until the vegetables are cooked through, soft and starting to char slightly.

Preheat the grill on a medium–high setting.

Remove the tray from the oven, add the halloumi and tomatoes, then transfer the tray to the grill and cook for 7–10 minutes, until the halloumi is golden.

Meanwhile, for the parsley yogurt dressing, mix the yogurt and parsley together in a small bowl.

Serve the tray bake with dollops of parsley yogurt dressing, garnished with chopped parsley and sprinkled with smoked paprika.

1 red pepper, cut into large
   chunks
1 yellow pepper, cut into
   large chunks
1 courgette, cut into large
   chunks
½ head of broccoli, cut into
   small florets
1 red onion, cut into large
   wedges
4 garlic cloves, peeled
5 teaspoons harissa
2 tablespoons lemon juice
glug of olive oil
400g (14oz) can chickpeas,
   rinsed, drained and patted dry
1 lemon, quartered
250g (9oz) halloumi cheese,
   cut into 12 cubes
3 tomatoes, quartered

For the parsley yogurt dressing:
6 tablespoons Greek yogurt
1½ tablespoons chopped flat
   leaf parsley

To garnish:
chopped flat leaf parsley
1 teaspoon smoked paprika

PIMP IT UP POST-WORKOUT

Cook 50g (1¾oz) brown rice per person. Dish up your veg and halloumi and, before serving, add the rice to the baking tray and give it a quick mix so it soaks up some of the juices in the tray.

BABA'S BEEF KOFTE
WITH CREAMY TAHINI
#FAISALFAKEAWAY

My Dad's kofte recipe comes all the way from Egypt. It was handed down by his mother and it always reminds me of home when I eat it. I remember Dad spending hours in the kitchen preparing feasts for us, and his kofte was his speciality. He rolls them out and cooks them over the barbecue whatever the weather, but I grill or fry mine, because I don't have a garden. (Sob!) This dish provides a great hit of protein and healthy fats but, more importantly, it tastes delicious.

First, make the tahini sauce. Put all the ingredients, excluding the seasoning and measured water, into a bowl and mix with a spoon until a thick sauce develops. Slowly mix in the water until you reach a consistency you like. Season with salt and pepper. Set aside in the refrigerator.

To make the koftes, put the onion, garlic and parsley into a food processor and pulse until everything is finely chopped and the juices of the onions are oozing out. The mixture should look nice and green. Add more parsley if it doesn't. Transfer the mixture to a large bowl and add the remaining kofte ingredients, excluding the oil. Massage together for a few minutes until well mixed. Cover with clingfilm and refrigerate for at least an hour or overnight if possible.

Heat the oil in a frying pan or griddle over medium heat. While the pan is heating, divide the kofte mixture into 16 portions and roll each one into a small sausage roughly 8cm (3¼ inches) long. Place them on a plate and square off the sides so you can turn them easily in the pan and cook all sides evenly.

Cook the koftes for about 6 minutes (1½ minutes on each side) or until cooked through. Then increase the heat to high and cook for about 2 minutes, turning occasionally, until lightly charred, to get the barbecue effect. Remove from the pan and leave to rest for 5 minutes before serving.

Garnish your koftes with chopped curly parsley and serve them with a drizzle of the creamy tahini sauce and my fresh Feta Salad (see page 160), if liked.

PIMP IT UP POST-WORKOUT

Serve your meal with a wholemeal pitta or my Freakin' Fast Flatbreads (see page 182 – just omit the coconut) to make a delicious kofte sandwich, or use the bread to mop up the leftover tahini on your plate.

1 large white onion, roughly chopped
2 garlic cloves, peeled
2 large handfuls of curly parsley, plus extra if needed
500g (1lb 2oz) beef mince (or use a half-half mixture of lamb and beef mince)
3 teaspoons ground cumin
1 teaspoon smoked paprika
2 teaspoons paprika
1 teaspoon ground black pepper
large pinch of salt
drizzle of olive oil

Feta Salad (see page 160) to serve (optional)
chopped curly parsley, to garnish

For the tahini sauce:
3 tablespoons tahini
4 tablespoons lemon juice
2 teaspoons cider vinegar
2 teaspoons ground cumin
1½ teaspoons garlic powder
2–3 tablespoons lukewarm water
salt and pepper, to taste

TIP:

Double or triple your quantities, then freeze the uncooked meat mixture. Whenever you fancy this dish, defrost the mixture thoroughly, then shape and cook it as described.

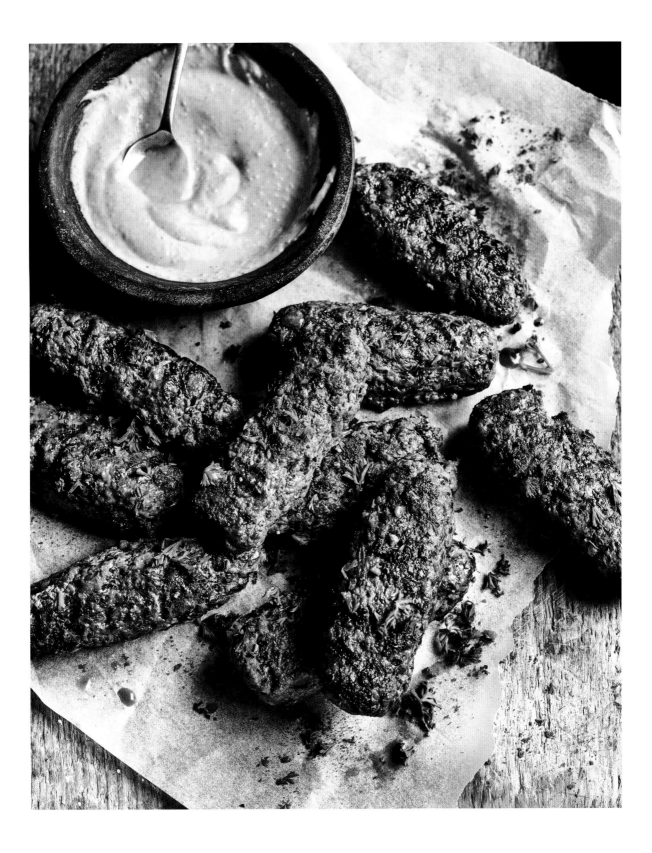

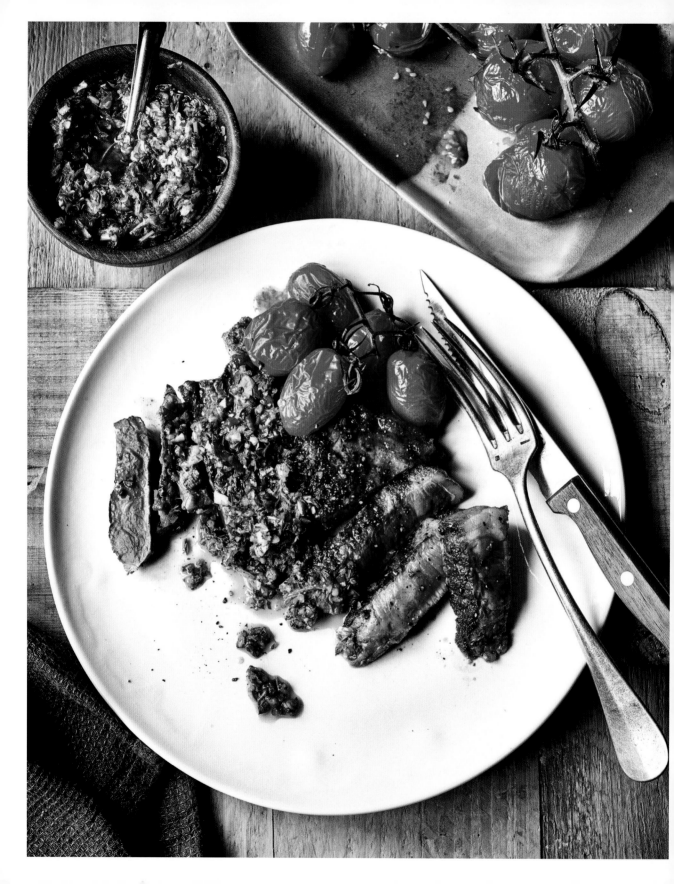

STEAK CHIMICHURRI WITH ROASTED VINE TOMATOES

SERVES 4

Argentinian Chimichurri sauce never lasts long in our house! Drizzle it over steak and you might struggle to eat steak again without it.

Preheat the oven to 200°C (400°F), Gas Mark 6. Remove your steaks from the refrigerator so they have about 20 minutes at room temperature before cooking.

To cook the tomatoes, put the vines into a baking dish, drizzle over the olive oil and season with salt. Cook for 12–15 minutes, until soft and juicy.

While the tomatoes are cooking, make the chimichurri sauce. Throw all the ingredients, excluding the vinegar and oil, into a food processor and whiz them up. Transfer to a bowl and mix in the vinegar, then pour over the oil to cover the mixture. Leave the sauce to sit while you prepare your steak.

Set a frying pan over high heat and heat the pan until very hot (do not grease it). Meanwhile, sprinkle the salt, pepper and garlic granules over both sides of the steak and drizzle with olive oil. Gently massage the oil and seasoning into the meat. Now put the steaks into the pan. Fry the steaks for about 2 minutes on each side for medium–rare, depending on the thickness of the steaks, and 4–5 minutes on each side for well done – do not move the steaks except when you flip them over. Remove from the pan and leave to rest for 5 minutes, then slice and serve with the chimichurri spooned over the juicy steaks and the roasted-on-the-vine tomatoes alongside.

PIMP IT UP POST-WORKOUT

Steak and chips is always a winner. Try serving this post-workout with Crispy Parsnip Chips (*see* page 181) or Sweet Potato Chips (*see* page 190).

#MEATFREEMONDAY

For a vegetarian option, substitute portobello mushrooms for the steaks (2 per person.) Destalk and slightly hollow out the mushrooms before cooking in the oven for 10 minutes at 200°C (400°F), Gas Mark 6. Meanwhile, fry the hollowed-out mushroom scraps for 2 minutes in a drizzle of olive oil with a crushed garlic clove and a pinch of chilli flakes before wilting 50g (1¾oz) baby spinach in the pan. Drain the mushroom juices. Add the spinach mixture to 40g (1½oz) of mashed garden peas and 20g (¾oz) of crumbled feta before stuffing the mushrooms and cooking for a further 5 minutes and serving with the chimichurri sauce.

4 sirloin steaks, about 195g (6¾oz) each
2 pinches of salt
2 large pinches of ground black pepper
2 large pinches of garlic granules
1 tablespoon olive oil

For the tomatoes:
24—32 tomatoes on the vine
drizzle of olive oil
salt, to taste

For the chimichurri sauce:
2 garlic cloves, peeled
2 tablespoons chopped oregano
2 large handfuls of curly parsley
1 large handful of fresh coriander leaves
¼ teaspoon dried chilli flakes
½ red onion
good pinch of fine sea salt
good pinch of ground black pepper
2 tablespoons red wine vinegar
3—4 tablespoons extra virgin olive oil

TIP:

You can refrigerate your chimichurri sauce for up to 2 days. Just make sure you bring it back to room temperature before you serve it.

EDGWARE ROAD CHICKEN TAOUK WITH MINT YOGURT AND FETA SALAD #FAISALFAKEAWAY

SERVES 4 (MAKES 8 SKEWERS)

I am half Egyptian and half Irish and, as most Egyptians in London will tell you, Edgware Road is the place to go if you want a cracking kebab. The street comes alive at night, and the restaurants churn out the taste of home from their hot coals. I almost always order a chicken taouk, which is chicken marinated in yogurt and spices and skewered. Here is my version – it's great for lunch or dinner.

Throw the diced chicken into a freezer bag with the remaining ingredients and rub it all together through the bag so it is thoroughly mixed. Place the bag in the refrigerator and leave to marinate for a few hours if you can.

When ready to cook, prepare a barbecue or preheat the grill on a high setting. Skewer the chicken pieces onto metal skewers or pre-soaked bamboo skewers. Aim for about 4 chicken pieces per skewer. Barbecue for about 10 minutes or grill for 12–15 minutes, turning every few minutes, until the chicken is cooked through (the juices run should clear when the meat is pierced with a knife).

While the chicken is cooking, make the mint yogurt. Mix all the ingredients in a bowl, garnish with smoked paprika and set aside until ready to serve.

To make the feta salad, put all the ingredients into a bowl and mix.

Serve the chicken skewers with the mint yogurt and feta salad alongside.

PIMP IT UP POST-WORKOUT

Make a little wholemeal sandwich with some Freakin' Fast Flatbreads (*see page 182*) – just substitute the spices for whatever you fancy.

#MEATFREEMONDAY

For a vegetarian version of this dish, substitute halloumi and vegetables for the chicken. Use 300g (10½oz) halloumi, 1 red pepper, 1 yellow pepper, 1 red onion, 1 courgette – all evenly cubed and skewered after marinating. Lightly grease a grill pan with a little rub or spray of olive oil, and place the skewers on the tray. Cook under a hot grill for 10–12 minutes, turning halfway through, until the vegetables have softened and the cheese has turned golden.

For the chicken:
6 chicken breasts (about 900g/2lb), evenly diced
1 teaspoon smoked paprika
1 teaspoon dried oregano
1 teaspoon sumac
2 teaspoons dried thyme
2 teaspoons garlic powder
2 teaspoons tomato purée
1 tablespoon cider vinegar
2 tablespoons olive oil
5 tablespoons Greek yogurt
4 tablespoons lemon juice
pinch of salt
pinch of ground black pepper

For the mint yogurt:
8 tablespoons Greek yogurt
little-finger-sized length of cucumber, peeled and grated
1 teaspoon garlic powder
4 sprigs of mint, leaves very finely chopped
pinch of salt
pinch of ground black pepper
smoked paprika, to garnish

For the feta salad:
6 tomatoes, roughly chopped
1 small cucumber, roughly chopped
100g (3½oz) feta cheese, diced
glug of extra virgin olive oil
pinch of ground black pepper

TIP:

I quadruple the dried spice mix quantities and store the mixture in an old spice jar labelled "taouk".

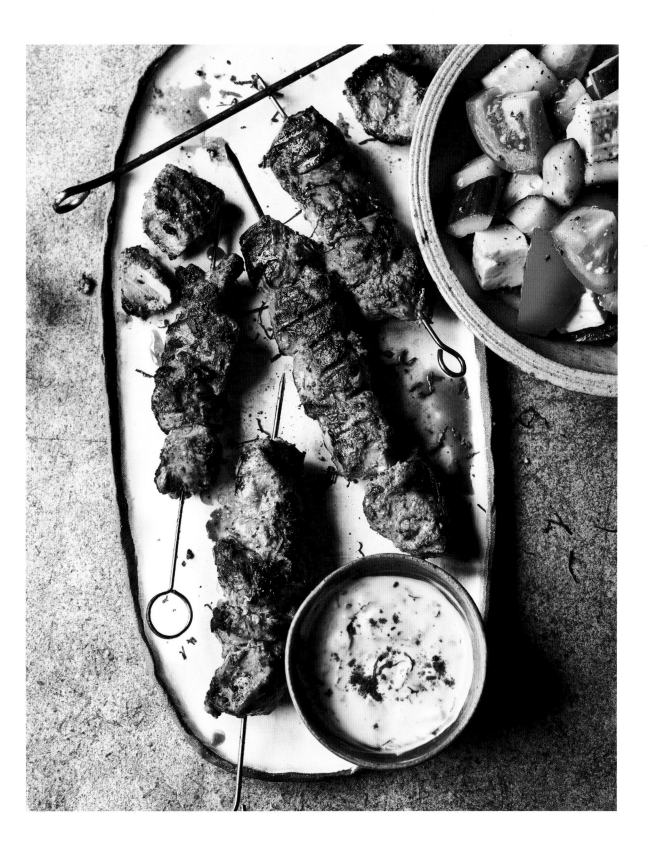

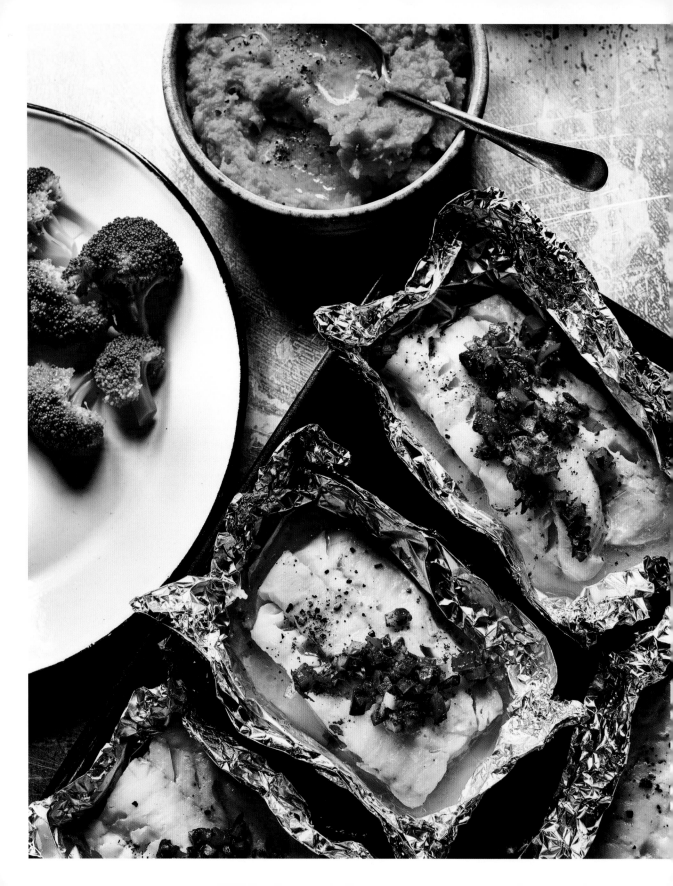

BUTTERY BAKED COD
AND EZME SALAD

I first tried ezme salad while holidaying in Turkey a few years ago. It's a delicious salad, and I love it with baked cod. Its fresh, spicy tang with the flaky, buttery fish is a match made in heaven. And it takes only 15 minutes to cook – this dish is an all-round winner! Get your greens in by serving it with steamed or roasted broccoli.

Preheat the oven to 180°C (350°F), Gas Mark 4.

Lay a large rectangle of kitchen foil on your work surface and place a cod fillet in the centre. Place a knob of butter on the fish and a little black pepper. Seal the parcel very loosely around the fish and place it on a baking tray. Repeat with the remaining cod fillets.

Bake for about 15 minutes until the fish is opaque and flakes easily with a fork.

While the fish is cooking, make the ezme salad. Mix all the ingredients in a large bowl and leave to sit for at least 10 minutes.

Serve the cod immediately with the ezme salad spooned over the fish or alongside it, accompanied by the broccoli.

PIMP IT UP POST-WORKOUT

Serve this with some Garlic Sweet Potato Mash. Peel and dice 2 sweet potatoes and boil for about 20 minutes, until tender. Drain well. Put a knob of butter, 2½ tablespoons almond milk and 2 teaspoons garlic powder into a saucepan set over a gentle heat. Once the butter is melted, return the sweet potatoes to the pan and mash well. Serve sprinkled with freshly ground black pepper.

#MEATFREEMONDAY

For a vegetarian version of this dish, preheat oven to 200°C (400°F), Gas Mark 6. Cut the tops off 4 green peppers to create lids and core and deseed. Stand on a baking tray. Sauté 8 chopped spring onions, 2 crushed garlic cloves and 300g (10½oz) spinach on a medium–low heat for about 1 minute until the leaves are wilted. Mix the spinach mixture thoroughly in a big bowl with 1 tablespoon milk, 2 beaten eggs and 60g (2¼oz) pine nuts and then divide between the peppers. Replace the tops and bake for 35–40 minutes, until the skins are soft and wrinkly. Serve immediately with the ezme salad.

4 cod fillets, about 140g (5oz) each (or use haddock), skinned and boned
4 knobs of butter
couple of pinches of ground black pepper
steamed or roasted broccoli, to serve

For the ezme salad:
3 plum tomatoes, deseeded and finely chopped
½ red onion, very finely diced
½ red pepper, very finely diced
4 teaspoons finely chopped black olives
1½ teaspoons sumac
2 generous pinches of chilli flakes
4 tablespoons finely chopped flat leaf parsley
2 teaspoons red wine vinegar
4 tablespoons extra virgin olive oil
salt and pepper, to taste

TIP:

This dish is just as good for lunch as it is for dinner. If you are feeling lazy, put the foil parcels with the cooked fish onto plates, tip your ezme salad into the foil parcels and save yourself some washing up. It combines so well with the buttery juices from the cod. If you have a barbecue, make up a load of ezme and top your meat with it to avoid the temptation of the sugar-laden shop-bought sauces.

ROASTED CAULIFLOWER AND CHICKPEA TURMERIC SALAD #MEATFREEMONDAY

Turmeric is having a bit of a moment, thanks to its widely reported health benefits, and it's a really versatile ingredient. This salad is a Meatfree Monday favourite of mine, with chickpeas providing a nice punch of protein and creamy tahini ticking the good fats box. The sweet crunchy burst of pomegranate seeds breaks up the rich creaminess of the tahini, so don't scrimp on them.

Preheat the oven and a large, deep baking tray to 200°C (400°F), Gas Mark 6.

In a large bowl, toss the cauliflower and chickpeas in the oil, cumin, fennel and turmeric. Pour the mixture into the preheated baking tray and spread it out in a single layer. Bake for 15–20 minutes, until the cauliflower begins to soften and brown. Stir the contents of the baking tray to give everything a turn, then return it to the oven and bake for another 15–20 minutes, until the chickpeas have crisped up and the cauliflower is golden brown all over.

Stir the onion into the tray and roast for a further 5–10 minutes, until the onion has softened, taking care not to burn your veg.

Put the kale into a large bowl, add enough of the tahini sauce to coat the leaves, then massage the dressing into the leaves well. (Any leftover sauce can be refrigerated and drizzled over meat or veg the next day.) Leave to stand for 5 minutes, then mix in the contents of the baking tray, straight from the oven.

To serve, squeeze over the orange juice, which brings out the flavour of the tahini, and garnish with pomegranate seeds.

1 cauliflower, broken into small florets
400g (14oz) can chickpeas, rinsed, drained and patted dry
2 tablespoons olive oil
1 tablespoon ground cumin
1 teaspoon fennel seeds
1 tablespoon ground turmeric
½ red onion, sliced
3 large handfuls of kale, destalked and torn into small pieces
up to 1 quantity Tahini Sauce (*see* page 156)
juice of 1 orange
2 handfuls of pomegranate seeds, to garnish

PIMP IT UP POST-WORKOUT

Za'atar-roasted Sweet Potatoes work nicely mixed in with this dish. Dice a washed, unpeeled sweet potato, pop it onto a baking tray and toss the dice in 2 teaspoons coconut oil. Bake in a preheated oven, 200°C (400°F), Gas Mark 6, for 5–10 minutes before you put the tray with the cauliflower and chickpeas into the oven. Later, give the sweet potato a turn when you turn the cauliflower. Then, when you add the onions to the cauliflower, sprinkle 2 teaspoons za'atar over the sweet potato. Remove from the oven with the cauliflower and add to the kale.

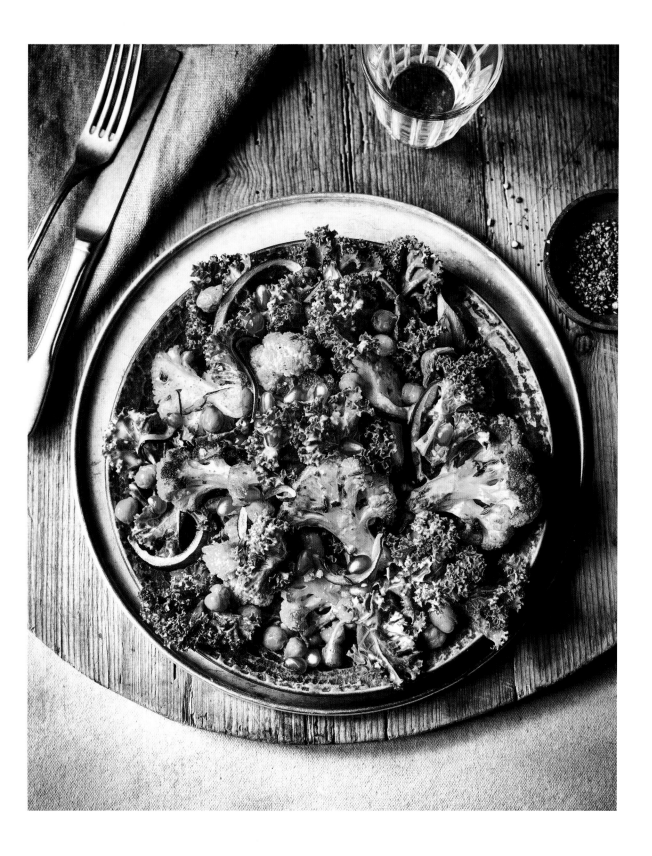

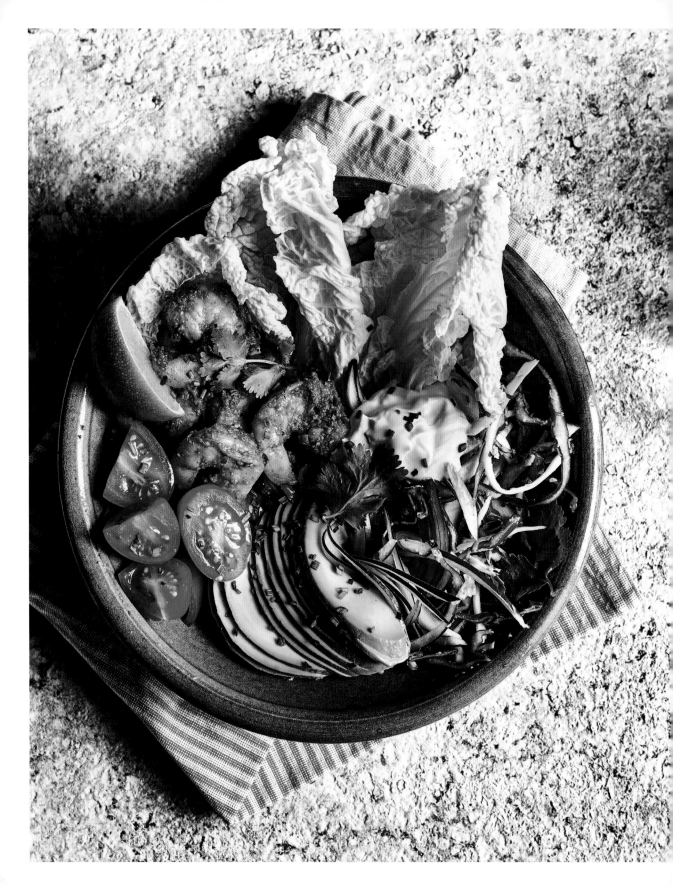

PRAWN TACO BOWLS WITH ZINGY SLAW

SERVES 4

These super-tasty taco bowls are great for lunch or dinner, quick to assemble and need barely any cooking time. I've gone for prawns here but you can use beef, veggies, tofu or chicken instead, and salad ingredients of your choice. I've provided a spice blend recipe that makes more than you need, but it keeps well in an airtight container, so you can use it each time you fancy this dish.

First, make the spice blend. Put all the ingredients into an empty jar, screw on the lid and give the jar a good shake.

Put the prawns into a bowl and put the peppers into another bowl. Add 1½ tablespoons spice blend to the prawns and 1½ tablespoons, along with a splash of olive oil, to the peppers. Mix to ensure everything is well coated. Cover and leave to marinate for about 20 minutes if you have time.

While your taco mix is marinating, put all the ingredients for the slaw, except the shredded cabbage, into a blender and whiz them up until smooth. Set aside.

Fry the peppers in a frying pan over medium heat for 3–5 minutes, until they begin to soften, then add the prawns and cook for about 2 minutes, until the prawns are cooked. Stir the lime juice into the hot pan.

Mix your shredded cabbage into the slaw mixture just before serving.

Divide the tomatoes, avocado, onion and lettuce between 4 bowls, then divide your pepper-and-prawn mixture as well. Top each bowl with 1 tablespoon Greek yogurt, some chopped chives and a good handful of zingy slaw and garnish with a lime wedge for squeezing over.

PIMP IT UP POST-WORKOUT

Cook 30–40g (1–1½oz) brown rice per person. Rinse and drain a 400g (14oz) can of black beans. Heat up the beans in a saucepan over medium–low heat for 3–4 minutes, until they are warmed through but not mushy. Share the rice and beans between the 4 bowls.

#MEATFREEMONDAY

Substitute 400g (14oz) tofu, cut into strips, for the prawns.

For the spice blend:
8 teaspoons garlic granules
6 teaspoons ground coriander
8 teaspoons paprika
8 teaspoons ground cumin
4 teaspoons dried coriander
4 teaspoons cayenne pepper
4 pinches of chilli flakes
4 small pinches of salt
4 pinches of pepper

For the taco bowl:
400g (14oz) raw peeled and
    deveined king prawns
2 mixed peppers of your colour
    choice, sliced
3 tablespoons spice blend
    (see above)
glug of olive oil
juice of ½ lime
3 tomatoes, chopped
2 avocados, sliced
½ red onion, sliced
4 Chinese lettuce leaves

For the zingy slaw:
2 tablespoons chopped fresh
    coriander, plus extra
    to garnish
5 spring onions
2 garlic cloves
½ teaspoon ground cumin
zest and juice of 1 lime
glug of extra virgin olive oil
½ white or red cabbage, shredded

To garnish:
4 tablespoons Greek yogurt
handful of chopped chives
lime wedges

TANDOORI PRAWNS
WITH RAITA SLAW
#FAISALFAKEAWAY

SERVES 3-4

Bursting with flavour, these juicy prawns are packed full of protein and omega 3 fatty acids, and are also a great source of iron, zinc and vitamin E. I normally just cook them in a pan and serve them up with all their juices on a bed of spinach, but they are also delicious threaded onto skewers and barbecued. Wolf them down with some crunchy, minty raita-style slaw.

Combine the ingredients for the spice blend in a bowl and mix well.

Place your prawns in a freezer bag with the yogurt and tomato purée. Add the spice blend and mix thoroughly in the bag - massage the mixture through the bag to keep your hands clean. Leave in the refrigerator to marinate for at least 20 minutes, or overnight if possible.

Combine all the ingredients for the slaw, except the cabbage, in a blender until smooth. Set aside.

To cook, heat the oil in a frying pan set over medium heat. Add the prawns. If you're using precooked prawns, they just need heating through for about 2 minutes. Raw prawns will take a little longer but will be juicier - they will be cooked and pink within 3-6 minutes, depending on their size. In the final 30 seconds of cooking, stir in the lemon juice.

Mix the shredded cabbage into the slaw mixture just before serving.

Serve the prawns and all the juices over a bed of uncooked spinach. Garnish with fresh coriander, if you have any to hand, and serve with the slaw alongside.

For the spice blend:
1 teaspoon ground ginger
1 teaspoon ground cumin
1 teaspoon ground coriander
1 teaspoon cayenne pepper
1 teaspoon salt
1 teaspoon ground nutmeg
1 teaspoon garlic powder
1½ teaspoons paprika
a few saffron strands (optional)

For the prawns:
300g (10½oz) raw or cooked, peeled and deveined king prawns
3 tablespoons Greek yogurt
1 teaspoon tomato purée
1½ teaspoons coconut oil
2 tablespoons lemon juice
2 large handfuls of spinach
fresh coriander leaves, to garnish (optional)

For the raita slaw:
¼ cucumber
2 garlic cloves, peeled
handful of mint leaves
½ handful of fresh coriander
½ teaspoon ground cumin
1 teaspoon maple syrup
2 tablespoons Greek yogurt
½ white cabbage, shredded
¼ red cabbage, shredded (or use extra white cabbage)
salt and pepper, to taste

PIMP IT UP POST-WORKOUT

My Freakin' Fast Flatbreads (*see* page 182) work perfectly with this dish. Alternatively, cook up 50g (1¾oz) brown rice per person.

ZESTY ZA'ATAR COD WITH BROCCOLI COUSCOUS

Za'atar is a Middle Eastern spice blend that I have a habit of sprinkling on almost everything – blame the Egyptian in me! It works so well with buttery fish. The broccoli "couscous" has a pleasing crispiness to it. Add crunchy pistachio, feta and pomegranate and it makes a tasty and very colourful accompaniment for the fish.

Rub a drizzle of olive oil on both sides of your cod fillets, then sprinkle ½ teaspoon za'atar over each side of each fillet.

Heat 2 teaspoons olive oil in a large frying pan over high heat. When it is nice and hot, add your fillets and fry for 2–3 minutes on each side, or until the fish is cooked through – it should be opaque, flaky and lightly golden.

Meanwhile, melt the ghee or coconut oil in a frying pan over medium heat. Put the grated broccoli into a bowl and stir in the garlic granules, black pepper and salt, then tip it into the frying pan and stir for about 3 seconds to coat it in the ghee or oil. Stir in the pistachios and measured water. Cover the pan with a lid or kitchen foil and cook for 1–2 minutes, until the raw edge is taken off the broccoli, but it has not become soggy or mushy.

Transfer to a bowl and mix in two-thirds of the spring onion. Garnish with the crumbled feta, pomegranate and the remaining spring onion.

When the cod is cooked, transfer it to serving plates, then return the pan to the heat and melt the butter with the lemon juice, scraping any tasty bits off the pan and blending them into the mixture. When it is melted, drizzle 1 tablespoon over each fillet. Serve immediately, with the broccoli "couscous" alongside.

PIMP IT UP POST-WORKOUT

Add some Crushed Potatoes to get your carb fix. Allow 16–20 baby new potatoes (4–5 per person). Boil them until tender, then drain and crush roughly with a fork – you're looking to crush them, not mash them. Mix in 3 tablespoons lemon juice, 3 tablespoons extra virgin olive oil, 2 teaspoons chopped chives and 2 chopped spring onions and season with salt and pepper and you're ready to serve. Alternatively, substitute the broccoli for cooked quinoa.

For the cod:
- 2 teaspoons olive oil, plus a drizzle for oiling the fillets
- 4 cod fillets, about 140g (5oz) each
- 4 teaspoons za'atar
- 1 tablespoon butter
- 5 tablespoons lemon juice

For the broccoli couscous:
- ½ tablespoon ghee or coconut oil
- 1 head of broccoli, florets and stems coarsely grated
- 1 tablespoon garlic granules
- 1 teaspoon ground black pepper
- good pinch of fine sea salt
- 3 tablespoons chopped unsalted pistachios
- 2½ tablespoons water
- 3 spring onions, sliced

To garnish:
- 50g (1¾oz) feta cheese, crumbled
- 2 handfuls of pomegranate seeds

TIP:

My Ezme Salad (*see* page 163) goes well with this fish.

INCREDIBLE HULK
MISO SALMON BOWL

SERVES 4

I call this an Incredible Hulk bowl because it is bursting with green gains, not because it makes me angry when I eat it! The miso dressing and salmon flaked through the greens is an absolute dream. Please, please make this so you know what I mean. I'm probably not allowed to have a favourite recipe, but if I were…

Preheat the oven to 200°C (400°F), Gas Mark 6.

Grease a baking tray, then arrange the salmon fillets in it, skin-sides down. Bake for 12–15 minutes or until cooked through and flaking easily. Transfer to a plate and leave to cool.

Bring a saucepan of water to the boil. Add the green beans and boil for 2 minutes. Now add the broccoli florets and boil for 2 minutes more, until the broccoli and green beans are crisp-tender. Drain under running cold water, then transfer to a bowl and cover with cold water to halt the cooking process. Leave to cool, then drain.

To make the dressing, combine all the ingredients, excluding the lime juice, measured water and olive oil, in a bowl. Mix well until any lumps have dissolved and you have a smooth paste, then add the remaining ingredients and continue mixing until thoroughly blended. Set aside.

Cut the portion of cucumber in half along its length and use a spoon to scoop out and discard the watery seeds. Chop it and put it into a bowl with the spring onion, spinach, spiralized courgette, coriander and chives. Add the cooled beans and broccoli to the bowl and give everything a good mix. Pour in the dressing and mix again.

Flake the cooled salmon into the salad and gently mix it through. Sprinkle with the sesame seeds, then serve.

PIMP IT UP POST-WORKOUT

Cook 40g (1½oz) buckwheat noodles per person according to the packet instructions. Drain and rinse under running cold water to cool, then put them into a bowl and mix in a drizzle of extra virgin olive oil to prevent them sticking together. Mix them in with the salad ingredients when they are cold.

For the miso dressing:
1½ tablespoons miso paste
1 teaspoon soy sauce
1 teaspoon rice wine (mirin)
1 teaspoon balsamic vinegar
1 teaspoon sesame oil
½ teaspoon ground ginger
½ teaspoon garlic powder
3 teaspoons lime juice
2 tablespoons water
1 teaspoon extra virgin
   olive oil

For the salad:
olive oil, for greasing
3 salmon fillets, about 130g
   (4½oz) each
100g (3½oz) fine green beans
½ head of broccoli, broken
   into florets
½ cucumber
3 spring onions, finely sliced
3 handfuls of spinach leaves
½ courgette, spiralized
1 tablespoon finely chopped fresh
   coriander (optional)
1 tablespoon finely chopped
   chives (optional)
large pinch of sesame seeds

TIP:

If you don't own a spiralizer, run the length of the courgette down the larger-bladed side of a grater in one movement to create long, grated strands. Discard the seedy core.

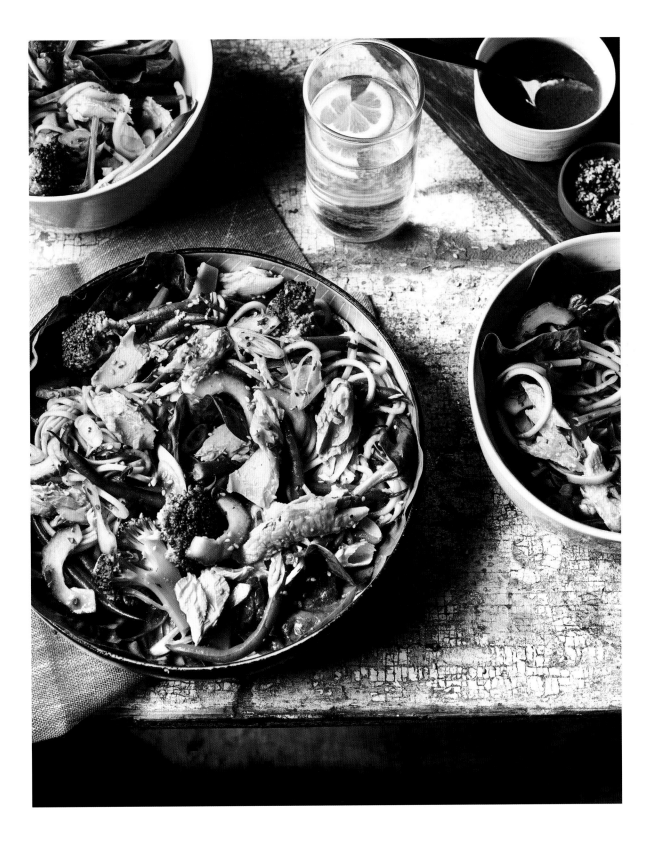

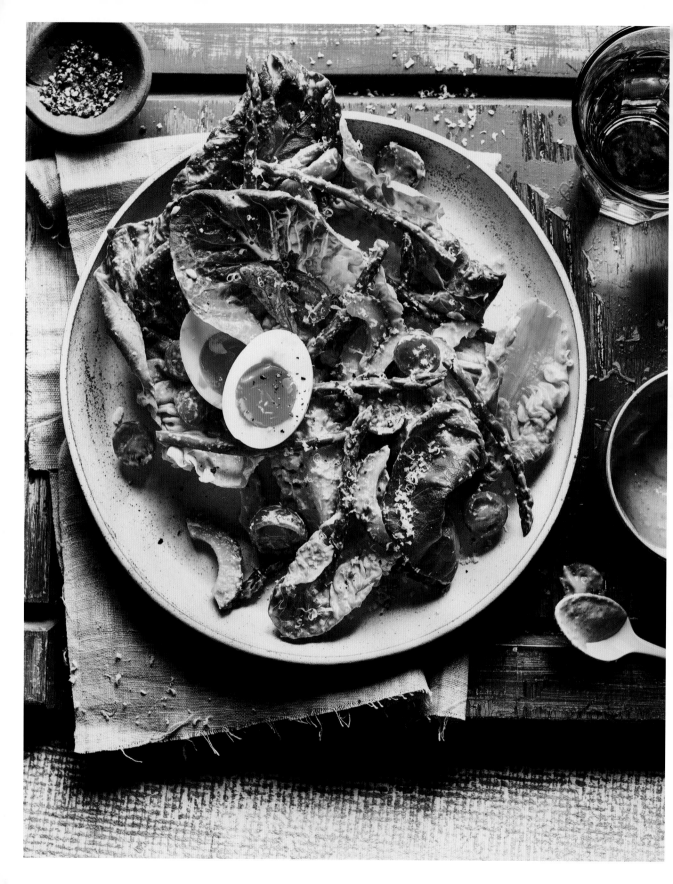

CAESAR SALAD GOES GREEN
#MEATFREEMONDAY
#FAISALFAKEAWAY

Caesar salad is one of my favourite salads, but the rich, creamy dressing makes it one to avoid when I eat out. I decided to make a healthier version to enjoy at home, using a little avocado and Greek yogurt to create the creaminess. By swapping anchovies for capers to recreate that salty tang, this salad is a great one for Meatfree Monday or vegetarians.

To make the dressing, put all the ingredients into a blender and blend until smooth. Set aside.

Bring a saucepan of water to a boil. Carefully lower in the eggs and boil for 6-7 minutes. Transfer the eggs to a bowl of cold water to halt the cooking process and make them easier to shell.

Steam the asparagus spears for about 5 minutes, or until tender. Leave to cool.

Halve the cucumber portion along its length, then scoop out the seeds with a spoon and discard (removing the seeds allows the cucumber to remain crisp). Chop the deseeded cucumber, then put it into a large bowl with the tomatoes, lettuce and cooled asparagus. Pour in half the dressing and mix well. Now taste the salad and add more dressing if desired. Divide the salad into 4 portions and transfer them to bowls.

Shell and halve the eggs, then add them to the bowls. Sprinkle over some grated Parmesan, then grind over some black pepper and serve immediately.

For the dressing:

¼ avocado

2½ teaspoons capers

4½ tablespoons Greek yogurt

2 teaspoons Dijon mustard

10g (⅓oz) Parmesan cheese, grated

2 tablespoons cider vinegar

2 garlic cloves

2 tablespoons extra virgin olive oil

3 tablespoons water

For the salad:

4 eggs

20 fine asparagus spears

½ cucumber

16 cherry tomatoes, halved

4 large handfuls of crisp lettuce, such as Cos or Romaine

ground black pepper

grated Parmesan cheese, to garnish

PIMP IT UP POST-WORKOUT

Croutons are the obvious choice when it comes to Caesar salad, but they are dripping in oil, and there is already enough oil in the dressing. Fake it by cubing up a slice of rye bread each and sprinkling it through your salad.

TIP:

The eggs and yogurt here provide you with lots of good protein, but if you really want to add chicken, you can. I sometimes shred up leftover roast chicken and add it to the salad when I make it the next day.

DINNER

MISO SALMON WITH SESAME PAK CHOI

SERVES 4

Miso is a traditional Japanese seasoning made from fermented soy beans which is packed with protein and makes everything you add it to taste phenomenal. It pairs perfectly with fish.

First, marinate the salmon. Put the miso paste, mirin, vinegar, soy sauce, maple syrup, the ginger and garlic powders and 1 teaspoon of the sesame oil into a bowl and stir to blend to a smooth paste. Transfer to a freezer bag, add the salmon fillets and seal. Gently massage to coat the fish with the marinade inside the bag. Refrigerate for a minimum of 20 minutes, or overnight if possible.

When ready to cook, preheat the oven to 200°C (400°F), Gas Mark 6.

Drizzle the groundnut oil and the remaining sesame oil across a baking tray. When the oven is hot, lay the salmon fillets, skin-sides down, in the prepared tray and bake for about 15 minutes or until the fish is flaky and cooked through.

Meanwhile, prepare the pak choi. Cut the base off each head of pak choi to separate the leaves. Discard any leaves that have gone soggy.

Heat the oil in a saucepan over medium heat, then add the garlic, chilli flakes and pak choi. Toss the leaves around until they are coated with oil, then reduce the heat to low, add the water and cover the pan with a lid. Simmer for 2 minutes, shaking the pan occasionally so the leaves don't burn, then add the sesame seeds and soy sauce. Simmer for 3–4 minutes or until the pak choi is cooked.

Serve the fish garnished with spring onions, if using, and the pak choi alongside.

For the miso salmon:
- 2½ tablespoons miso paste
- 1 tablespoon rice wine (mirin)
- 2 teaspoons balsamic vinegar
- 1 tablespoon soy sauce
- 1 teaspoon maple syrup
- ½ teaspoon ground ginger
- ½ teaspoon garlic powder
- 2 teaspoons sesame oil
- 1 teaspoon groundnut oil
- 4 salmon fillets, about 130g (4½oz) each
- 2 spring onions, sliced, to garnish (optional)

For the sesame pak choi:
- 3 heads of pak choi
- 2 teaspoons sesame oil
- 1 garlic clove, crushed
- pinch of dried red chilli flakes
- 2 teaspoons water
- 2 teaspoons sesame seeds
- 1½ teaspoons soy sauce

PIMP IT UP POST-WORKOUT

Keep it simple with a side serving of brown rice (cook 50g/1¾oz per person), or cook and cool your brown rice, then turn it into egg-fried rice by following the instructions on pages 188–9.

#MEATFREEMONDAY

Substitute aubergine for the fish. Cut 2 large aubergines in half, score the pale flesh so the marinade can sink in, then marinate for about 30 minutes. Place the aubergines in the tray, cut-sides down, and bake at 200°C (400°F), Gas Mark 6 for about 25 minutes, or until softened.

MRS PMA'S THAI TURKEY BURGERS WITH ALMOND BUTTER SATAY SAUCE #FAISALFAKEAWAY

SERVES 4

If you're craving a Thai takeaway, stop! These fragrant turkey burgers are nice and lean, with a subtle kick that will leave your tummy feeling very happy – so step away from the phone. The satay sauce, made with almond butter and coconut milk, is so good it's almost drinkable, plus it stays fresh for a couple of days so you can keep going back for more – which you will, because this recipe is so damn good! Serve your burgers and satay sauce with some steamed broccoli spears or mangetout.

To make the burgers, put all the ingredients, except the mince and coconut oil, into a food processor and whiz until everything is finely chopped and blended. (You can do this by hand, but it adds on a lot of prep time.)

Transfer the mixture to a large bowl, add the turkey mince and mix well. I like to do this by hand and mash the chopped mixture into the meat, so it is evenly blended. You can cook these immediately if you want, but I recommend you cover the bowl with clingfilm and refrigerate for 30 minutes, or overnight if possible, to enhance the flavours.

When you're ready to cook, shape the meat into 8 patties straight from the refrigerator – the colder the mixture is, the easier it is to mould.

You'll cook the patties in 2 batches of 4. Heat ½ teaspoon of the coconut oil and ¼ teaspoon of the sesame oil in a large frying pan over medium heat. Fry the patties for about 3 minutes on each side, or until the burgers are cooked through and the juices run clear. Leave the burgers to rest for 5 minutes before serving.

Meanwhile, make the satay sauce. Put all the ingredients into a blender and whiz up until smooth.

Serve the burgers garnished with spring onion and some chopped coriander and chilli, with the satay sauce on the side or drizzled over.

PIMP IT UP POST-WORKOUT

Serve with brown rice. Cook roughly 50g (1¾oz) rice per person, then stir through some toasted desiccated coconut and chopped fresh coriander before serving.

For the turkey burgers:
½ Scotch bonnet chilli, deseeded
thumb-sized piece of fresh root ginger, peeled and grated
5 spring onions
3 garlic cloves
2 tablespoons chopped chives
1 tablespoon chopped fresh coriander
2½ tablespoons soy sauce
zest and juice of 1 lime
1 tablespoon sesame oil, plus ½ teaspoon for cooking
500g (1lb 2oz) lean turkey mince
1 teaspoon coconut oil

For the satay sauce:
1 tablespoon soy sauce
1 tablespoon sesame oil
1 tablespoon maple syrup
5 tablespoons almond butter
juice of 1 lime
6 tablespoons coconut milk
¼ Scotch bonnet chilli, deseeded
2 garlic cloves
1 spring onion
½ thumb-sized piece of fresh root ginger, peeled and chopped

To garnish:
shredded spring onion
chopped fresh coriander
chopped chillies

TIP:

Make extra burger mixture for the freezer. Defrost thoroughly and mould your burgers whenever you fancy this dish.

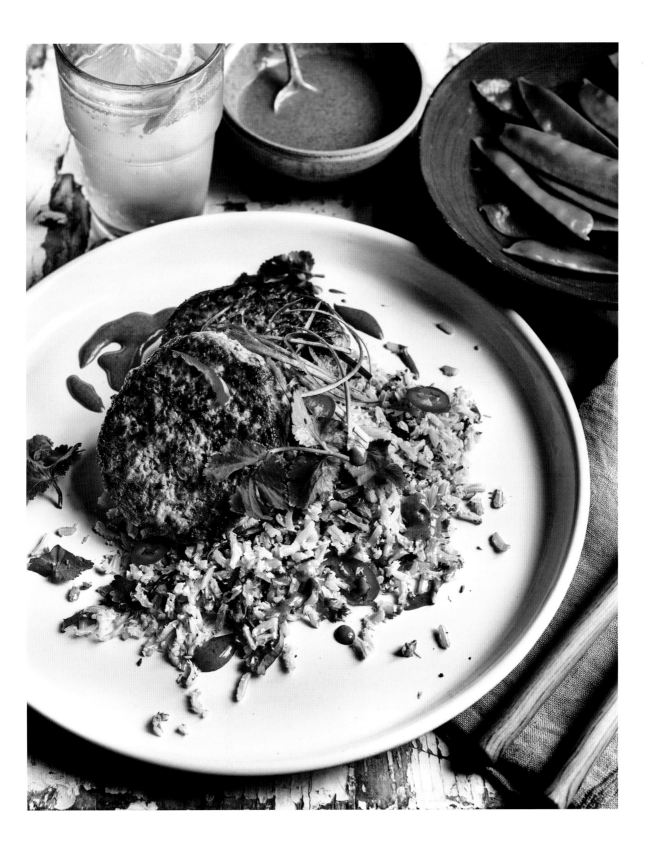

SPICY MEATBALLS WITH CRISPY KALE

SERVES 3-4

These meatballs are kept lean by using turkey mince (but feel free to substitute another meat) as it is low in fat and calories, but high in protein, which is essential for muscle growth and repair. It's also high in vitamin B6, a cheeky little vitamin for fighting fatigue. I serve mine with Crispy Kale because I love the contrast in textures and because kale is one of the most nutritious foods on the planet, but these juicy meatballs are also awesome paired with "courgetti". (*See* page 193 for a quick courgette spaghetti recipe.)

Preheat the oven to 200°C (400°F), Gas Mark 6. Pop in a roasting dish to heat up.

Whack all your meatball ingredients, excluding the oil, into a large bowl and mix well by hand. Mould the mixture into 18 meatballs of even size.

Heat the oil in a frying pan over medium heat. Sear the meatballs for 5 minutes, until they form a golden crust all over, then remove from the pan and set aside.

Use the same pan to make your sauce, so it takes on all the meat juices. Put the onion and red pepper into the pan and fry over medium heat for about 3 minutes, until the onion begins to soften. Add the garlic granules and herbs and mix it all together. After 30 seconds, add your chopped tomatoes, spinach, passata, pepper and measured water and stir again.

Transfer the mixture to the preheated roasting dish, add the meatballs and give it all a good mix to ensure your meatballs are covered in the thick sauce. Add more water at this stage if you prefer a runnier tomato sauce, as it will reduce further in the oven. Bake for 10–15 minutes, until the sauce is thick, reduced and bubbling away and the meatballs are cooked through.

Meanwhile, put the kale into a bowl, drizzle in some olive oil and mix so the leaves are very lightly coated. Arrange the leaves on a large baking tray, being careful not to overcrowd it, and sprinkle with the fine sea salt. (I've kept them plain here as there's a lot of flavour going on with the meat, but in other dishes you can use coconut oil or add paprika, garlic granules, cayenne pepper, ground cumin, chilli flakes, you name it.)

For the spicy meatballs:
450g (1lb) turkey mince (2 per cent fat)
2 garlic cloves, crushed
thumb-sized piece of fresh root ginger, peeled and grated
1 red onion, finely diced
1 egg
1 tablespoon soy sauce
2 teaspoons Worcestershire sauce
1 tablespoon English mustard (or use 1 teaspoon mustard powder)
1 teaspoon ground cumin
1 teaspoon smoked paprika
1 teaspoon paprika
1 teaspoon chilli flakes
1 tablespoon chopped fresh coriander, plus extra to garnish
2 teaspoons olive oil
grated Parmesan cheese, to garnish

For the tomato sauce:
1 white onion, diced
1 red pepper, diced
2 teaspoons garlic granules
1 teaspoon oregano
1 teaspoon thyme
large pinch of ground black pepper
400g (14oz) can chopped tomatoes
2 handfuls of spinach leaves
6 tablespoons passata
2 tablespoons water, plus extra as desired

Add the tray to the oven when the meatballs have been in for roughly 5 minutes, and bake for 9-11 minutes or until the leaves are crispy, turning them over halfway through the cooking time to prevent burning. They should be browning at the edges but not burnt, and will continue to crisp up once out of the oven. Keep an eye on them as they turn quite quickly - although I quite like the nuttiness when they are slightly burnt.

Put the roasting dish on a heatproof plate on your table and serve the meatballs from the dish, with a sprinkling of grated Parmesan, garnished with coriander, and the kale alongside.

For the crispy kale:
4 large handfuls of chopped
   kale, destalked and torn into
   bite-sized pieces
glug of olive oil
good pinch of fine sea salt

TIP:

The meatball mix here can also be used to make spicy turkey burgers and makes 7-9 patties. Shape the mixture into patties, then fry for a few minutes on each side until browned, about 5-7 minutes, and finish in the oven at 200°C (400°F), Gas Mark 6 for 10-12 minutes or until cooked through. If you double your quantities when you make this, you can split the mixture in half before moulding, to make burgers and meatballs from one batch.

PIMP IT UP POST-WORKOUT

Serve this dish with wholemeal spaghetti - just don't overdo it as it's easy to cook too much. About 50g (1¾oz) per person should do the trick.

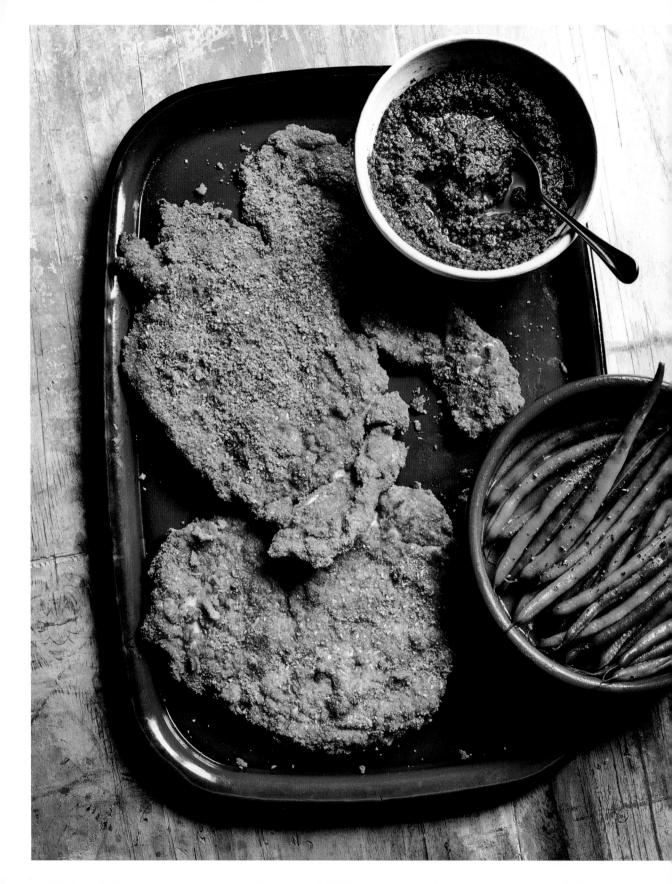

CHICKEN ESCALOPE WITH LEMON-BUTTER GREEN BEANS

I use ground almonds to create the crisp on this chicken, so you get extra protein and don't need to deep-fry your meat like fast food chain restaurants do. Serve with my garlicky walnut pesto.

Preheat the oven to 220°C (425°F), Gas Mark 7. Drizzle the olive oil or ghee into a deep baking tray and pop this into the oven to heat up. Put each chicken breast into a freezer bag or between 2 sheets of clingfilm and bash them into thinner chicken steaks using a rolling pin or the base of a pan.

Put the ground almonds, garlic granules, onion powder, smoked paprika and cayenne pepper into a bowl. Set this on your work surface next to a bowl containing the whisked egg. Dip each chicken steak first into the egg, then into the almond mixture to coat it. Arrange the coated chicken steaks in the preheated baking tray. Bake for 15 minutes, then turn and bake for another 10 minutes, or until the chicken is cooked through.

Meanwhile, prepare the beans. Bring a saucepan of water to a boil, then boil or steam the beans for 4–5 minutes. Drain and set aside. Return the pan to the hob, add the butter and lemon juice and melt the butter over low heat. Add the pepper and garlic, then return the beans to the pan and toss until the beans are well coated. Serve immediately alongside the chicken and Walnut Pesto.

PIMP IT UP POST-WORKOUT

Add my Crispy Parsnip Chips – they can be cooked in the oven with the chicken at 220°C (425°F), Gas Mark 7. Warm a roasting tin in the oven. Peel 500g (1lb 2oz) parsnips and cut them into evenly sized chips. Boil for 3 minutes to soften slightly, then drain. Transfer to a bowl, add 2 teaspoons mustard powder, 1 teaspoon paprika, 1 teaspoon dried rosemary and 3 tablespoons polenta and toss well to coat. Arrange in the roasting tin and roast for 30-40 minutes, turning halfway through, until cooked and crispy.

#MEATFREEMONDAY

Substitute a 400g (14oz) block of firm tofu for the chicken. Drain the block. Put some sheets of kitchen paper on a plate, then place the block on top. Place a few more sheets of kitchen paper over the tofu block, then place an upturned plate over it. Place a weight on top and leave for 10 minutes to remove the water. Slice the block into 4 x 100g (3½oz) steaks. Coat it as described above, then bake at 220°C (425°F), Gas Mark 7 for 30 minutes, turning it 3 times.

1½ teaspoons olive oil or ghee

4 chicken breasts, about 160g (5¾oz) each

150g (5½oz) ground almonds

2 teaspoons garlic granules

2 teaspoons onion powder

2 teaspoons smoked paprika

¼ teaspoon cayenne pepper

2 eggs, whisked

Walnut Pesto (see page 184), to serve (optional)

For the lemon-butter green beans:

4 handfuls of green beans

1½ tablespoons butter

2 tablespoons lemon juice

1 teaspoon ground black pepper

2 pinches of garlic granules

TIP:

You can reheat this chicken, but it is best to do so in a frying pan to regain some of the crisp.

MRS PMA'S CAULIFLOWER AND PANEER COCONUT CURRY #MEATFREEMONDAY #FAISALFAKEAWAY

SERVES 4-5

This is a Meatfree Monday favourite of mine, and makes a great Saturday night Fakeaway, too. It is fragrant and delicate, with a gentle kick, and it smells ridiculously good. Serve it with Crispy Kale (see pages 178–9) or Egg-fried Cauliflower Rice (see pages 188–9). If you are eating this post-workout, mop up the juices with some super-simple Freakin' Fast Flatbreads (see below). Hell, yeah!

Heat 1 tablespoon of the oil in a saucepan over medium heat. Add the paneer and aubergine and cook for 3-4 minutes, until the paneer is golden and the aubergine begins to colour and soften. Transfer to a bowl and set aside.

Heat the remaining oil in the same pan, then add the dry spices and seeds and cook for about 1 minute, until fragrant. Stir in the cauliflower and onions, ensure they are coated, then add the ginger, chilli and garlic. Cook for about 1½ minutes.

Stir in a splash or two of the coconut milk. Wait another minute, then add the remaining coconut milk and the coconut water, adding extra water as desired if you like the sauce thinner. Cook for about 10 minutes, stirring occasionally.

Mix in the spinach along with the reserved aubergine and paneer, and cook for a further 5 minutes, until the sauce thickens slightly. The aubergine should soften in this time but still have a bit of a bite to it. Stir in the lime juice for the final minute of cooking.

Before serving, scatter over a handful of chopped coriander.

PIMP IT UP POST-WORKOUT

Try my Freakin' Fast Flatbreads. Put 160g (5¾oz) wholemeal self-raising flour into a bowl with 7 tablespoons Greek yogurt, 1 teaspoon garlic powder, 1 teaspoon nigella seeds, 2 teaspoons dried coriander and 2 teaspoons desiccated coconut. Bring together with your hands to form a dough. Dust the work surface with flour, then knead the dough for 3-5 minutes. Divide into 4 balls and cover with a clean tea towel until ready to cook. Then heat 1 teaspoon coconut oil in a large frying pan. Roll out each ball of dough into a disc. Fry for about 2 minutes on each side, until golden. Serve immediately.

3 tablespoons groundnut oil
200g (7oz) paneer, diced
1 aubergine, diced
2 teaspoons ground turmeric
2 teaspoons garam masala
1 teaspoon curry powder
1 teaspoon ground cumin
½ teaspoon cumin seeds
½ teaspoon mustard seeds
½ teaspoon fennel seeds
1 small head of cauliflower, cut into small florets
1 white onion, sliced
thumb-sized piece of fresh root ginger, peeled and grated
1 red chilli, deseeded and finely chopped
2 garlic cloves, grated
200ml (7fl oz) canned coconut milk
4—5 tablespoons coconut water, plus more as desired
2 handfuls of spinach leaves
juice of 1 lime
handful of roughly chopped fresh coriander, to garnish

TIP:

Make the sauce ahead and freeze it – then you can cook whatever fresh vegetables or meat you want in it when you fancy a curry.

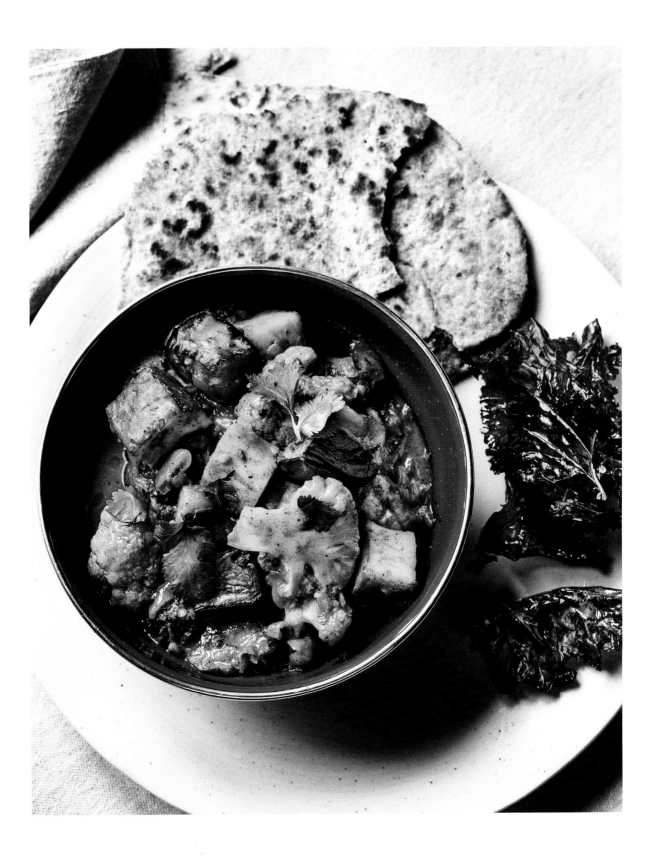

OH MY COD! LEMON COD WITH WALNUT PESTO AND ROASTED VEG

SERVES 4

I love how colourful this dish is. Fish is bursting with protein but can feel lighter than meat, which makes this one a good option when eating late after an evening workout. The walnut pesto is bursting with flavour and free from added preservatives. The recipe yields more pesto than you need for this dish, so you can freeze the excess or refrigerate it to use over the following days.

Preheat the oven to 190°C (375°F), Gas Mark 5.

To make the pesto, pulse the walnuts and garlic together in a food processor until the mixture resembles fine breadcrumbs. Add the remaining ingredients, excluding the oil, and pulse again as you slowly pour in just enough of the olive oil to achieve a nice pesto consistency. Pack the pesto into a clean jar and add a layer of olive oil to completely cover it. Set aside in the refrigerator. (Refrigerate for up to 5 days.)

Put the broccoli into a roasting tin and drizzle it with olive oil. Roast for 7-10 minutes, mixing halfway, until the broccoli begins to soften.

Meanwhile, put the peppers, courgettes and onion into a bowl and mix with a glug of olive oil and the lemon juice, garlic granules, dried basil, pepper and chilli flakes.

Add the vegetables to the pan after your broccoli has cooked for 7-10 minutes and toss everything together. Roast for 10 minutes.

Arrange the tomatoes and fish fillets on top of the roasted vegetables. Place 1-2 teaspoons walnut pesto on each fillet, then top with a slice of lemon for an extra bit of zing. Reduce the oven temperature to 180°C (350°F), Gas Mark 4, and bake for 10-12 minutes, until the fish is cooked through and opaque. Serve garnished with basil leaves.

PIMP IT UP POST-WORKOUT

Cut a sweet potato into large dice and put these into the roasting tin first. Roast for 15-20 minutes, then add the broccoli and continue as above. Alternatively, brown rice or quinoa make lovely accompaniments. Cook 50g (1¾oz) per person.

For the walnut pesto:
100g (3½oz) walnuts
2-3 garlic cloves
15g (½oz) flat leaf parsley leaves
45g (1½oz) basil leaves
25g (1oz) Parmesan cheese, grated
3 tablespoons lemon juice
about 8 tablespoons extra virgin olive oil, plus a few glugs for the top of the jar
salt and pepper, to taste

For the cod:
2 handfuls of broccoli florets, roughly chopped
olive oil
1 yellow pepper, roughly chopped
1 orange pepper, roughly chopped
2 courgettes, roughly chopped
1 red onion, cut into small wedges
4 tablespoons lemon juice
1 teaspoon garlic granules
2 teaspoons dried basil
2 pinches of ground black pepper
pinch of chilli flakes
2 handfuls of cherry tomatoes
4 cod fillets, about 140g (5oz) each (or use haddock)
4-8 teaspoons walnut pesto (see above)
1 lemon, sliced
basil leaves, to garnish

TIP:

Freeze excess pesto in an ice cube tray. Little pesto cubes are great for when you need a little for soup, dressings or a frittata topping.

FINGER-LICKING STICKY CHICKEN
#FAISALFAKEAWAY

SERVES 3

I defy you to make your way through this meal without licking your fingers – or the plate, the spoon, the baking tray and anything else the sauce has touched! It really is finger-licking good. Serve it with some green beans, or try it with my Crispy Kale (*see page 178*) if you are craving a Chinese-style takeaway, and throw in some unsalted cashew nuts as it bakes. If you are eating this post-training, add some Chilli Lime Cobs to the mix (*see below*).

Preheat the oven to 200°C (400°F), Gas Mark 6.

Put the soy sauce, maple syrup, sesame oil, ginger powder, vinegar, onions, garlic and paprika into a medium bowl and mix until blended. Now add the chicken and massage the mixture into the meat to ensure it is well coated. Cover the bowl and leave in the refrigerator to marinate for 20 minutes if you can, or overnight, to maximize the flavour. (But don't worry if you don't have time – this dish is still spot on.)

Put the ghee or coconut oil into a deep baking tray. Arrange the chicken pieces in the tray, skin-sides up. Bake for 25 minutes, then remove the tray from the oven and spoon the juices over the meat to baste it.

Return the tray to the oven and bake for a further 10 minutes, then baste the meat with the juices again. Sprinkle over the sesame seeds.

Bake for another 10 minutes, until the chicken is cooked through (the juices should run clear when the meat is pierced with a knife), then increase the oven temperature to 240°C (475°F), Gas Mark 9 and bake for 5 minutes more to crisp up the skin. Serve immediately.

- 2 teaspoons soy sauce
- 3 teaspoons maple syrup
- ½ teaspoon sesame oil
- ½ teaspoon ground ginger
- 2 teaspoons cider vinegar
- 2 spring onions
- 1 teaspoon garlic powder
- 1 teaspoon paprika
- 6 skin-on and bone-in chicken thighs, about 150–160g (5½–5¾oz) each
- ½ tablespoon ghee or coconut oil
- ½ teaspoon sesame seeds

PIMP IT UP POST-WORKOUT

Chilli Lime Cobs work great with this dish. Boil 3 corn cobs in a large saucepan for 4–6 minutes, until cooked. Drain the cobs, then cut them into thirds using a sharp knife. Melt 1 tablespoon butter in a frying pan and add ½ deseeded and finely sliced red chilli and the juice of 1 lime. Fry the corn cobs in the flavoured butter for 1 minute, then serve alongside the chicken and greens with a handful of fresh coriander, if you have any to hand.

CHUNKY VEGETARIAN CHILLI
#MEATFREEMONDAY

SERVES 4

Don't rub your eyes after making this one because those jalapeños burn! This dish proves that vegetables are not boring. Reduce those tomatoey juices to a thick, sweet, rich sauce and enjoy this smoky, spicy chilli with chunky vegetables.

Heat 1 teaspoon of the oil in a frying pan over medium heat. Add the aubergine, courgette and mushrooms and cook for 5 minutes, until softened – not soggy. Transfer to a bowl and set aside.

Now heat the remaining oil in a large saucepan over medium–high heat. Add the onion, celery, peppers and garlic and cook for 5 minutes, until the onion starts to soften and become translucent. Add the jalapeño, chilli flakes, cumin, paprika and cinnamon and cook, stirring, for about 3 minutes, until the celery and peppers have softened.

Pour the chopped tomatoes into the pan, add the ground coriander, beans, 100ml (3½fl oz) of the vegetable stock and a pinch of sea salt. Bring to the boil, then simmer for 15 minutes, until the veg has cooked and the sauce has reduced a little.

Mix in the reserved aubergine, courgette and mushrooms, then simmer for a further 10 minutes, until the tomato sauce has reduced and thickened. If you would like it less thick, stir in more stock a tablespoonful at a time until you reach the desired consistency.

Serve garnished with the yogurt, grated cheese and chopped coriander with avocado chunks on the side.

2 teaspoons olive oil
1 aubergine, cut into large chunks
1 courgette, cut into large chunks
100g (3½oz) button mushrooms
1 white onion, diced
2 celery sticks, sliced
2 red peppers, roughly chopped
2 garlic cloves, crushed
1 jalapeño pepper, deseeded and finely diced
1 teaspoon chilli flakes
1 teaspoon ground cumin
1 teaspoon smoked paprika
1 teaspoon ground cinnamon
600g (1lb 5oz) canned chopped tomatoes
1½ teaspoons ground coriander
150g (5½oz) canned black beans (rinsed and drained weight)
up to 200ml (7fl oz) vegetable stock
pinch of salt

To serve:
4 tablespoons Greek yogurt
thumb-sized piece of Cheddar cheese, grated
handful of chopped fresh coriander
1 avocado, cut into big chunks

PIMP IT UP POST-WORKOUT

Serve your chilli on a roasted sweet potato. Preheat the oven to 190°C (375°F), Gas Mark 5. Wash the dirt from your sweet potato skins, then dab them dry with kitchen paper. Mix 1 teaspoon paprika with ½ teaspoon olive oil in a bowl. Rub the sweet potatoes with the mixture, then prick the skins a few times with a fork. Bake for 35–45 minutes or until cooked through.

TIP:

Blend any leftover chilli into a spicy vegetarian Mexican soup, adding more vegetable stock to thin it out. It is lovely post-workout with a chunk of wholemeal bread.

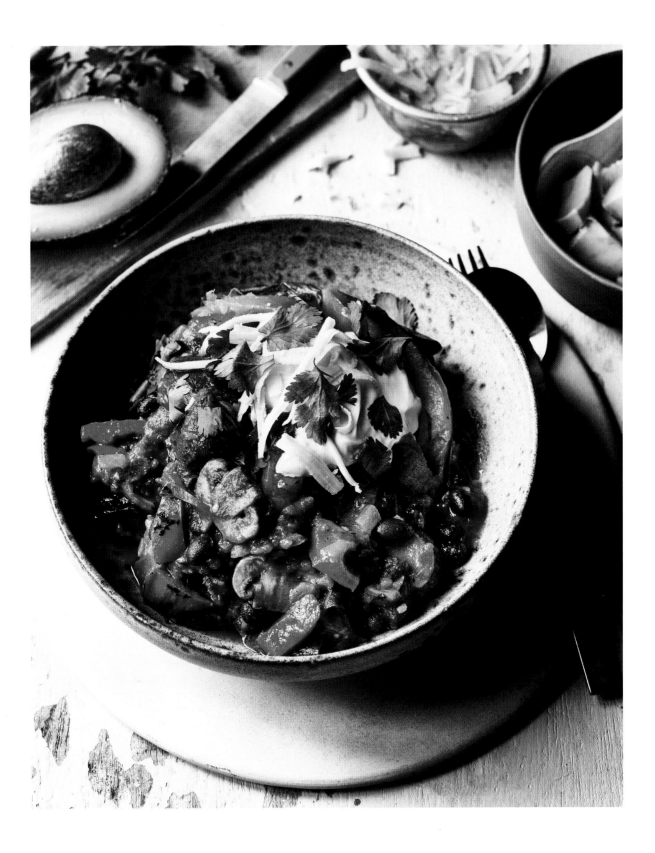

CHICKEN KATSU CURRY WITH EGG-FRIED CAULIFLOWER RICE #FAISALFAKEAWAY

SERVES 4

I'm a sucker for chicken katsu curry, so I had to master the curry sauce. Substituting ground almonds for the breadcrumbs keeps the carb content low, while the egg-fried cauliflower rice makes the meal even more saintly, and saves a huge amount of time in the kitchen. Batch-cook this sauce and you can have a tasty Fakeaway in no time during the week.

To prepare and cook the chicken, follow the method on page 181, leaving out the cayenne and paprika.

For the katsu sauce, melt the oil in a saucepan over medium heat. Add the carrots and onions and fry for about 5 minutes, until the onion softens and starts to become translucent.

Stir in the ginger and garlic and cook for 1 minute. Now stir in the gram flour, curry powder, turmeric and garam masala and add a little more oil if the mixture is dry and sticking to the pan. Then slowly stir in the stock – do not rush this process or the sauce might become lumpy.

Add the maple syrup, bay leaf and soy sauce and simmer for 20–25 minutes, until the carrots are nice and soft.

During the last 5 or so minutes of the cooking time for the chicken and sauce, make the cauliflower rice. Whisk the eggs, sesame oil and soy sauce together in a bowl and set side.

Heat the coconut oil in a frying pan over medium heat. Add the grated cauliflower and garlic powder and cook, stirring, for 2 minutes. Create a well in the centre of the mixture and pour in the reserved egg mixture as well as the spring onions, reserving a small handful for garnish. From the well, stir the mixture out into the "rice" to mix well. Sprinkle in some black pepper (don't be shy!). Cook for up to about a minute, stirring constantly, until the egg is cooked through. Remove from the heat.

Transfer to a serving plate and sprinkle over some coriander if you fancy, the toasted sesame seeds and the reserved spring onion.

For the chicken:
1½ teaspoons olive oil or ghee
4 chicken breasts, about 160g (5¾oz) each
150g (5½oz) ground almonds
2 teaspoons garlic granules
2 teaspoons onion powder
2 eggs, whisked

For the sauce:
1 tablespoon coconut or groundnut oil, plus extra as required
2 large carrots, finely diced
1 small white onion, finely diced
½ thumb-sized piece of fresh root ginger, peeled and grated
2 garlic cloves, crushed
3 tablespoons gram flour
1 tablespoon curry powder
1 teaspoon ground turmeric
1 teaspoon garam masala
400ml (14fl oz) chicken stock
1 tablespoon maple syrup
1 bay leaf
1 tablespoon soy sauce

For the egg-fried cauliflower rice:
3 large eggs
2 tablespoons sesame oil
2 tablespoons soy sauce
1 teaspoon coconut oil
1 head of cauliflower, grated
1 teaspoon garlic powder
4 spring onions, chopped
pinch of ground black pepper

Once the sauce is ready, remove the bay leaf and blend it all up until smooth. (If you don't have a blender, pass the sauce through a sieve.)

Slice the chicken diagonally and serve with the sauce poured on top and the cauliflower rice alongside.

`handful of chopped fresh coriander, to garnish (optional)`

`large handful of toasted sesame seeds, to garnish`

PIMP IT UP POST-WORKOUT

Substitute 50g (1¾oz) brown rice per person for the cauliflower (or a mixture of brown rice and quinoa) – it works best if the cooked rice is cold before you start to cook the egg-fried rice. Try throwing in a handful of edamame beans too – buy them frozen and add to the rice as you boil it for the last 5 minutes.

#MEATFREEMONDAY

Substitute a 400g (14oz) block of firm tofu for the chicken, and vegetable stock for the chicken stock. Follow the instructions with the #MeatfreeMonday option on page 181, omitting the cayenne pepper and paprika.

TIP:

This katsu sauce freezes well, so freeze leftover sauce, or make the sauce ahead of time and freeze it. You can also freeze your grated cauliflower and throw it into the pan straight from frozen. This will get you ahead and stops you wasting food whenever you don't need a whole cauliflower for a meal.

FISH AND CHIPS WITH MUSHY PEAS
#FAISALFAKEAWAY

The ultimate British takeaway goes under a healthy makeover here. No, it's not as good as the real thing, because greasy batter and vinegar-soaked chips are a national institution for a reason. But is a takeaway really worth it after all your hard training? This version certainly has its own merits, and will scratch the itch until your cheat day. Serve with some roasted tomatoes on the vine to substitute the ketchup!

To make the "batter" for your fish, mix the polenta, garlic powder, paprika, lemon zest and dill, if using, on a plate. Put the whisked egg in a shallow dish alongside this plate. Now dip your fish fillets in the whisked egg to cover them, then coat each fillet with the polenta crumb mix. Set aside.

Heat the olive oil in a frying pan over medium heat. When the pan is hot, add the fish and cook for about 2 minutes on each side (thicker fillets will require longer), until the fish is cooked through and the polenta is crispy.

Meanwhile, boil the frozen peas for about 2–3 minutes until cooked, then drain. Transfer to a bowl and mash well with a fork or potato masher, or pulse a few times in a blender, then stir in the yogurt, mint, chilli flakes and salt. Serve alongside the fish with lemon wedges for squeezing over.

For the fish:
7 tablespoons polenta
1 teaspoon garlic powder
1 teaspoon paprika
½ teaspoon chopped dill (optional)
finely grated zest of ½ lemon
1 egg, whisked
2 cod or haddock fillets, about 140g (5oz) each
glug of olive oil
lemon wedges, to serve

For the mushy peas:
150g (5½oz) frozen garden peas
3 teaspoons Greek yogurt
1½ teaspoon dried mint
pinch of chilli flakes
large pinch of salt

PIMP IT UP POST-WORKOUT

It is almost criminal to have fish and mushy peas without chips, so make sure you eat this after a workout so you can add my Sweet Potato Chips to your plate. A 250g (9oz) sweet potato will serve 2. Scrub it clean and pat dry. Cut off the end, then cut the potato into chips. Put them into a bowl with 1 tablespoon olive oil, 1 teaspoon paprika or ½ teaspoon smoked paprika, ½ tablespoon polenta, ¼ teaspoon cayenne pepper and ½ teaspoon garlic granules and mix well so the chips are lightly coated in the seasoned oil. Spread out on a baking tray - ensure they are not touching. Bake in the centre of a preheated oven, 200°C (400°F), Gas Mark 6, for 15 minutes, then flip them over and bake for a further 15 minutes, or until cooked through.

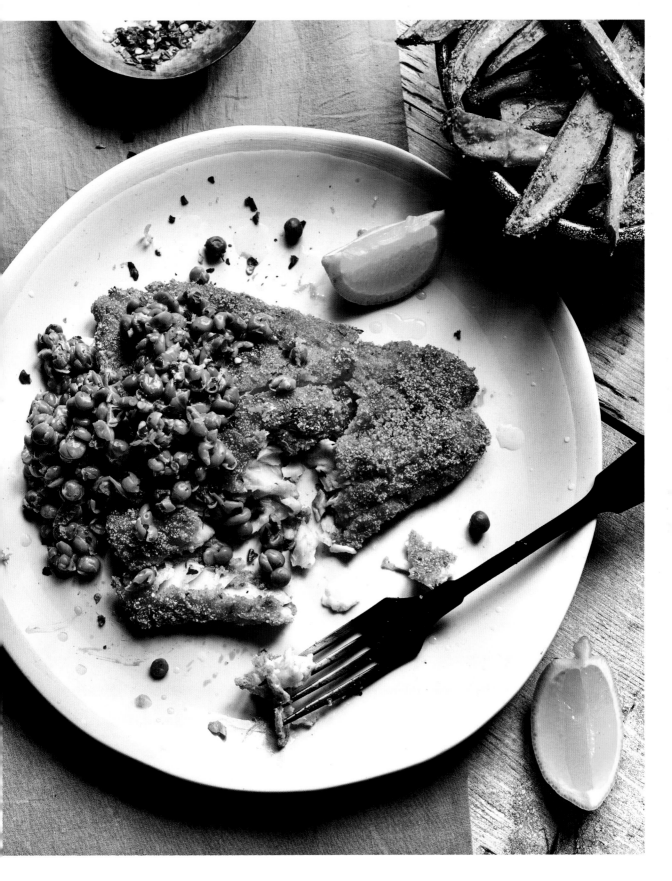

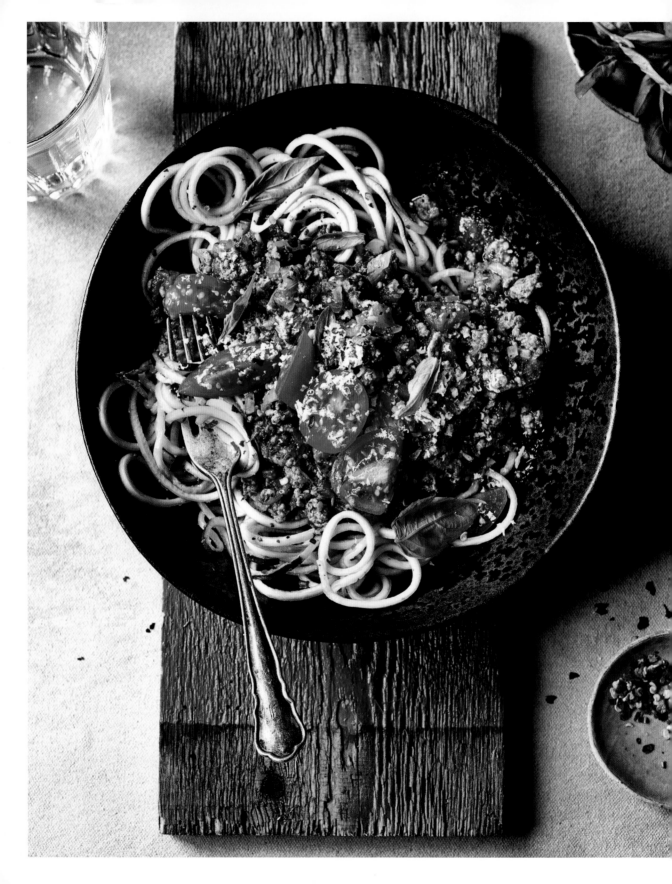

COURGETTI BOLOGNEASY

This is Bolognese with a healthy twist – courgette spaghetti, or "courgetti". When you fancy some comforting Italian food, it's a winner. Batch-cook the turkey Bolognese and freeze it in portions. You won't regret it. Once it's defrosted and heated through, you can make your courgetti in minutes. Easy peasy bologneasy!

To make the Bolognese, heat the coconut oil in a saucepan over medium heat. Add the turkey mince and cook for 3–4 minutes, until there are no pink bits left. Drain the juices and return the pan to the hob, then add the garlic, onion and celery. Fry for about 2 minutes, until the onion begins to soften.

Add the remaining Bolognese ingredients, adding the salt only if needed, and bring to a steady and vigorous simmer over medium to high heat. Once the sauce is bubbling away, reduce the heat to produce a low simmer and simmer for 15 minutes.

Meanwhile, prepare the courgetti. Spiralize the courgettes into spaghetti-like strands. If you don't have a spiralizer, repeatedly run the length of a courgette down the larger-bladed side of a grater in one movement to obtain long strands. Discard the seedy core. Set aside.

When the sauce looks ready, heat the oil in a frying pan over medium heat. Add the courgette and the remaining ingredients and fry for 1–3 minutes, until the courgette softens slightly.

Transfer the courgetti to serving plates, then serve the Bolognese sauce on a bed of courgetti, garnished with the cherry tomatoes and grated Parmesan. Add a few fresh basil leaves if you're feeling flash.

PIMP IT UP POST-WORKOUT

Serve with some healthy Garlic Flatbreads. Turn to page 182 and make my Freakin' Fast Flatbreads, without the added coriander, coconut, nigella seeds and garlic powder. Mix 150g (5½oz) salted butter, 2 crushed garlic cloves, 1 tablespoon chopped parsley and 1 tablespoon chopped chives in a bowl until the butter softens and everything is well mixed. Once the flatbreads are cooked, spread a little of the garlic butter on the breads to serve. Cover and refrigerate whatever butter you don't use, or freeze it in an ice cube tray, so it is portioned. Cover the tray with clingfilm before freezing.

For the Bolognese:
1 teaspoon coconut oil
450g (1lb) lean turkey mince
2 garlic cloves, crushed
1 white onion, finely diced
1 celery stick, finely diced
400g (14oz) can chopped tomatoes
1 teaspoon dried oregano
3 tablespoons dried basil
1 teaspoon ground black pepper
1 tablespoon Worcestershire sauce
1 teaspoon balsamic vinegar
pinch of salt (optional)

For the courgetti:
2–3 courgettes (1 per person)
1½ teaspoons olive oil
1 teaspoon garlic powder
pinch of salt
large pinch of pepper
pinch of chilli flakes (optional)

To garnish:
2 handfuls of cherry tomatoes or baby plum tomatoes, halved
grated Parmesan cheese
basil leaves (optional)

TIP:

Some supermarkets sell spiralized courgettes, but a spiralizer is a relatively cheap kitchen gadget and well worth the investment.

FIRE-ON-FIRE CHICKEN MADRAS
#FAISALFAKEAWAY

This is a thick, spicy chicken curry for those of you who like a bit of heat, and it cooks in less time than it takes for you to order a curry and have it arrive at your doorstep. The deep red colour from the chilli powder and tomatoes looks so inviting next to the green of the spinach and crunchy beans, while the coriander yogurt provides your tummy with some good fats... and your tongue with some relief.

Put the dry spices into a saucepan over medium–low heat and toast for about 1 minute, until they start to smell fragrant and jump in the pan. (If you aren't a fan of whole fragrant seeds in your curries, grind them after toasting using a pestle and mortar, then return to the pan.)

Add the ghee to the pan and stir it into the spices. Increase the heat to medium and add the ginger, garlic, chilli and onions. Stir until they are well coated in the spices, then add the diced chicken and coat it in the spices.

Cook for 2–3 minutes, stirring occasionally, until the chicken has turned white, then add the passata, mushrooms and bay leaf. Simmer, stirring frequently, for 20 minutes, until the curry has reduced to a thick sauce and the chicken is cooked through. (This is a thick curry, but if you prefer the sauce runnier, add a little chicken stock or water to loosen it.)

Meanwhile, bring a saucepan of water to a boil and boil the green beans for 3–4 minutes, until they are crisp-tender. Drain and set aside.

For the coriander yogurt, mix the yogurt and coriander together in a small bowl.

During the last 2 minutes of cooking the curry, add the beans and spinach to the pan and stir until all the spinach has wilted. Remove the bay leaf.

Serve with coriander yogurt and garnish with some red chilli slices and chopped fresh coriander, if liked.

PIMP IT UP POST-WORKOUT

Serve with Freakin' Fast Flatbreads (see page 182) or 50g (1¾oz) brown rice per person.

½ teaspoon ground ginger
½ teaspoon ground cumin
1 teaspoon fennel seeds
1 teaspoon cumin seeds
1 teaspoon ground cinnamon
1 teaspoon mustard seeds
1 teaspoon ground coriander
2 teaspoons garam masala
2–3 teaspoons hot chilli powder
1½ tablespoons ghee
thumb-sized piece of fresh root ginger, peeled and grated
3 garlic cloves, crushed
1 red chilli, finely diced
1 white onion, diced
4 chicken breasts, about 600g (1lb 5oz) total weight, diced
500g (1lb 2oz) passata
150g (5½oz) baby button mushrooms, halved
1 bay leaf
150g (5½oz) fine green beans, ends removed and halved
3 handfuls of spinach

For the coriander yogurt:
4 tablespoons Greek yogurt
handful of chopped fresh coriander

To garnish:
1 red chilli, sliced
chopped fresh coriander (optional)

TIP:

Mix it up and add different vegetables according to what you have in the refrigerator.

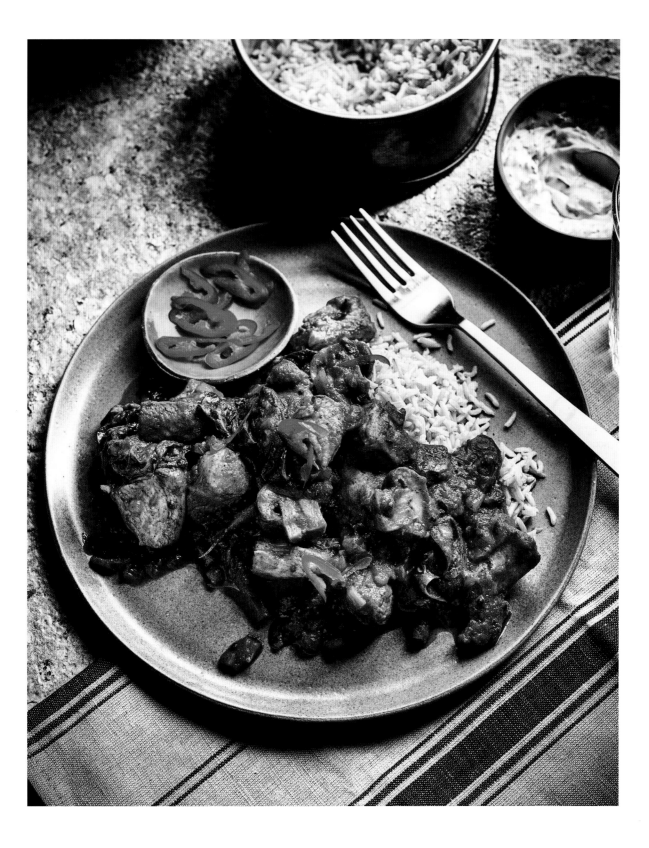

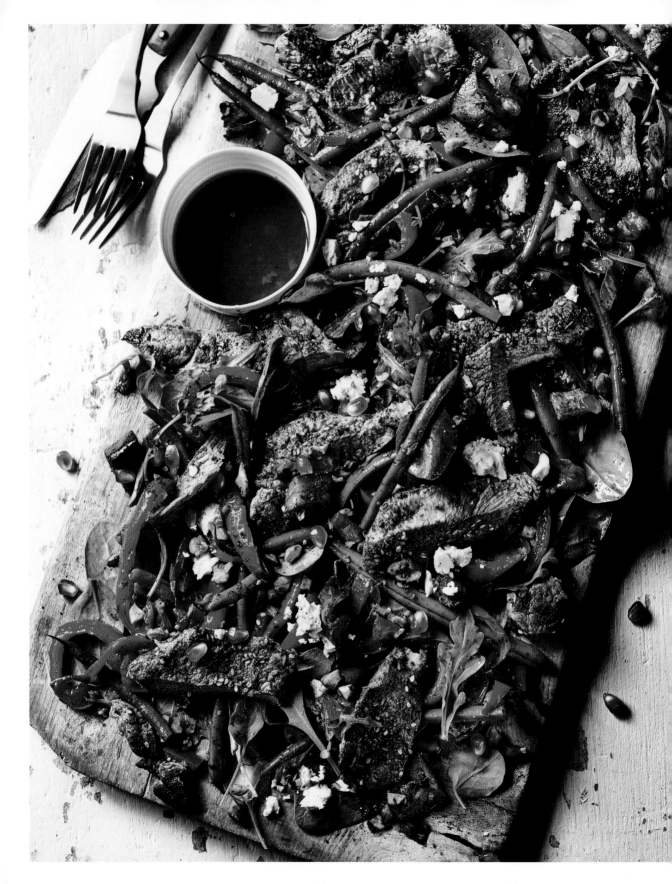

MIDDLE EASTERN LAMB STEAK SALAD

SERVES 4

I have a crush on this salad. It's herby, zesty, crunchy and meaty all at once! The juicy za'atar lamb with the crunch of the pistachios, the sweetness of the peppers, the creaminess of the feta, and the zing of the lemon and sumac amount to a salad-lover's dream. A fantastic quick dinner that you can throw together in no time.

Preheat the oven to 190°C (375°F), Gas Mark 5.

Put the peppers and aubergine on to a baking tray, drizzle over a little olive oil and season with salt. Roast for 20 minutes or until your peppers have started to soften and char slightly around the edges. If the aubergine needs slightly longer, leave it in for an extra 5 minutes.

Meanwhile, put the beans into a saucepan of water and bring to a boil, then simmer for 2 minutes, until crisp-tender. Drain the beans and place them in a bowl of cold water to halt the cooking process.

Drizzle each side of the lamb steaks with olive oil, then sprinkle with the za'atar.

Heat a frying pan over high heat, then add the steaks and cook for 1½–2 minutes on each side, until the meat is seared and browning slightly. I like to turn the steak and press the fatty edge onto the hot pan for about 30 seconds afterward, to brown it a little. Wrap the steaks in kitchen foil and leave to rest for 3–5 minutes.

To make the dressing, place all the ingredients in a jar and seal, and then shake until combined.

Mix the salad leaves with the pistachios, tomatoes, reserved beans, aubergine and red peppers, then add the dressing and toss (refrigerate any dressing you don't use for another day).

Crumble the feta over the salad, then roughly slice your lamb steaks and lay them on top of the salad. Add an extra little pinch of za'atar to finish.

PIMP IT UP POST-WORKOUT

Scoop your serving onto a wholemeal tortilla or pitta if you are feeling lazy, or add some Za'atar-roasted Sweet Potatoes to the salad (see page 164).

For the salad:
2 red peppers, sliced
1 aubergine, cut into bite-sized chunks
olive oil
200g (7oz) green beans
4 lamb steaks, about 95g (3¼oz) each
2 teaspoons za'atar, plus an extra pinch to garnish
4 large handfuls of mixed salad leaves
4 tablespoons roughly chopped pistachios
3 tomatoes, deseeded and roughly chopped
salt, to taste

For the dressing:
5 tablespoons extra virgin olive oil
grated zest and juice of 1 large lemon
1 tablespoon cider vinegar
2 garlic cloves, crushed
1 teaspoon paprika
2 tablespoons sumac
2 pinches of salt

For the garnish:
100g (3½oz) feta cheese
a small handful of pomegranate seeds, to garnish

TIP:

A handful of sliced radishes or some blanched, but still crunchy, cauliflower works well with this dish.

SNACK ATTACK

We all have days when the tummy starts growling long before dinner, especially when we are training hard. If you feel yourself getting those mid-afternoon munchies, my first piece of advice would be to drink some water. We often confuse thirst for hunger, so get some H_2O into the system. If you are still hungry, then of course you should eat a snack. Remember – don't fear food. If your body is telling you that you are hungry, it's because you are! Just snack smart – that means avoid the vending machine at all costs. If you prepare a little snack pack before leaving the house, you won't have to grab something unhealthy while you are on the go. Here are some of my favourite ways to shut up my stomach.

COTTAGE CHEESE PROTEIN POT

SERVES 2

Mix together the cheese, chives, smoked paprika and ground flaxseeds.

Gobble this up on top of a celery stick.

7 tablespoons cottage cheese
1 tablespoon chopped chives
¼ teaspoon smoked paprika
½ tablespoon ground flaxseeds

CAULIMOLE

SERVES 2

Boil the cauliflower until soft, then drain and cool under cold water. Transfer to a small bowl.

Add the remaining ingredients to the bowl and, using the back of a fork, mix and mash everything together.

This snack can be eaten with red pepper slices or cucumber batons.

½ head of cauliflower (about 4 florets), chopped
1 avocado
3 teaspoons lime juice
¼ teaspoon garlic granules
¼ teaspoon dried chilli flakes
½ teaspoon dried coriander

SCOTCH FLAX-EGGS

SERVES 4

As I've mentioned before, eggs are an absolute superfood in my book. They are a go-to snack of mine because they keep me full and stop me grazing on naughty things. These flaxseed-coated eggs give you an extra boost of good fats and protein while jazzing up the humble boiled egg and lending it a nice bit of texture. Add a bed of spinach and wedge of lemon to squeeze over and you are in snack heaven.

To cook the eggs, bring a saucepan of water to the boil, then reduce the heat to produce a quick simmer. Carefully lower in the eggs and simmer for 7 minutes, depending on the size of the eggs (you want a nice soft-set yolk). Cool in cold water, then shell the eggs.

Mix the paprika, salt and pepper with the flaxseed in a bowl. Roll each egg in the mixture.

Cut the eggs in half and place them in a little pot on a bed of spinach for a high-protein snack (1 egg per person). Add a little wedge of lemon if you like, and squeeze it over the egg before eating to give it a lift.

4 eggs
½ teaspoon smoked paprika
pinch of salt
pinch of pepper
2 tablespoons ground flaxseeds
40—50g (1½—1¾oz) spinach leaves
lemon wedges, to serve
    (optional)

TIP:

If you are struggling to make the coating stick, run the eggs under the tap and shake off the excess water before rolling.

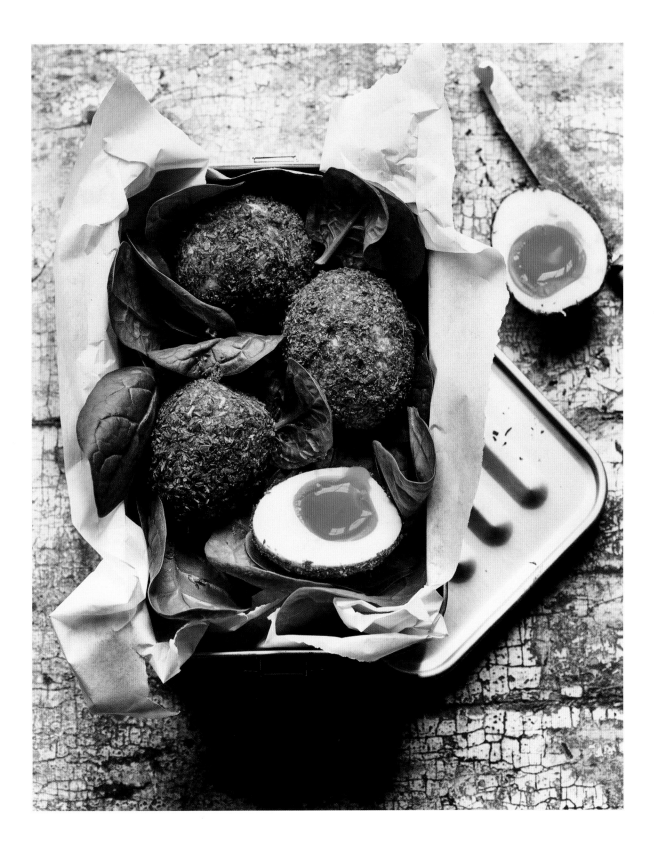

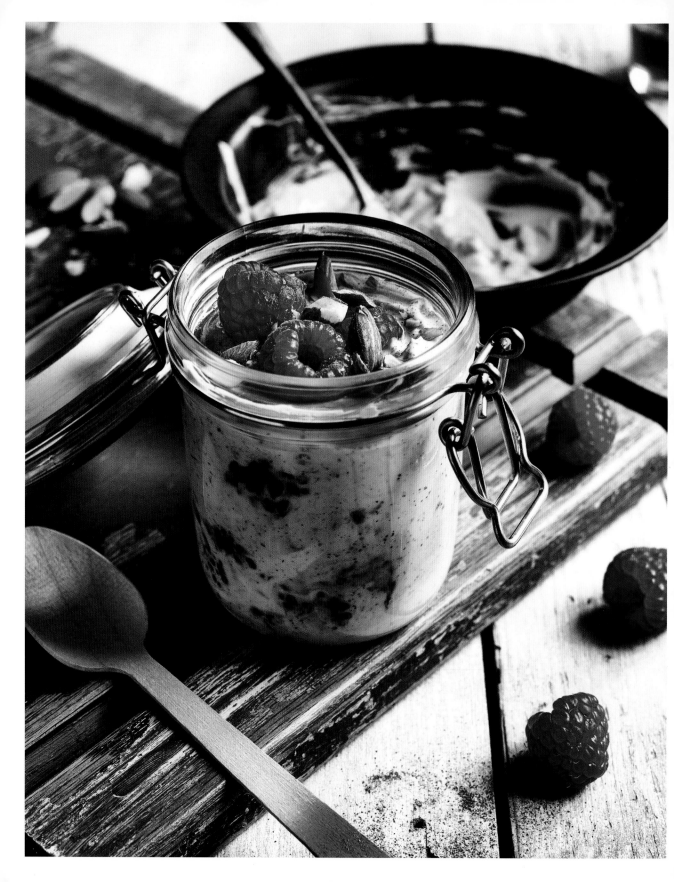

YOGGY POT

My yoggy pots really help me satisfy my sweet tooth when I get to that 4pm slump and feel a snack attack coming on. The beauty of them is that they are so easy to bung together and yogurt is a great, filling way to banish those tummy growls. Make up two or three days' worth of this at a time so you always have a healthy snack to hand if you need it.

Mix the ingredients together in a bowl, slightly mashing the raspberries as you go.

Decorate with extra raspberries and chopped almonds.

200g (7oz) Greek yogurt
1½ tablespoons chunky almond butter (look for brands containing nothing but nuts)
¼ teaspoon ground sweet cinnamon
¼ teaspoon maple syrup
10 raspberries, plus extra to decorate
chopped almonds, to decorate

CHEAT DAY

CHEESY SCOFFINS #CHEATDAY

MAKES 24

Is it a scone? Is it a muffin? No, it's a scoffin, and you will be scoffin' these in one sitting if you aren't careful! These wholemeal muffins with oozing pockets of melted cheese make a super-indulgent breakfast or mid-afternoon treat, without any nasty additives or hidden extras. The almond milk, Greek yogurt, wholemeal flour and olive oil serve as healthier substitutes and keep your scoffins lovely and moist. They are irresistible about 5 minutes after coming out of the oven. Cut them in half, spread with salted butter, sit back and enjoy.

350g (12oz) plain wholemeal flour
1 teaspoon salt
1 teaspoon bicarbonate of soda
1 teaspoon garlic powder
1 teaspoon onion powder
1½ teaspoons paprika
½ teaspoon mustard powder
150g (5½oz) Cheddar cheese, cut into very small dice
75g (2¾oz) Parmesan cheese, finely grated, plus 20g (¾oz) extra, for topping
4 spring onions, sliced
2 tablespoons chopped chives
100g (3½oz) Greek yogurt
200ml (7fl oz) almond milk
3 tablespoons olive oil, plus extra for greasing
2 eggs

Preheat the oven to 180°C (350°F), Gas Mark 4. Grease 2 x 12-hole muffin tins with olive oil.

Mix together the dry ingredients, Cheddar, Parmesan, spring onions and chives in a large bowl.

Whisk together the wet ingredients in a separate bowl.

Slowly add the wet mix to the dry mix, stirring it in with a spoon, until the mixture begins to come together. Once the dry mix starts to look wet, get in there with your hands and give it a good mix. The batter should feel lumpy and not too runny or wet.

Spoon the batter into the prepared muffin tins, filling each hole two-thirds full to allow space for the muffins to rise. Sprinkle the remaining grated Parmesan over the tops. Bake for about 25 minutes, until lightly golden.

Leave the muffins to cool in the tins for about 5 minutes, then remove from the tins and transfer to a wire rack to cool completely.

TIP:

Make a big batch and freeze the extra muffins. Separate each muffin with some baking paper and place in a sealable plastic container or a freezer bag. When cheat day comes around, just take out as many as you fancy and leave them for 30 minutes to defrost. Then bake at 180°C (350°F), Gas Mark 4 for 10 minutes to get that freshly baked feel.

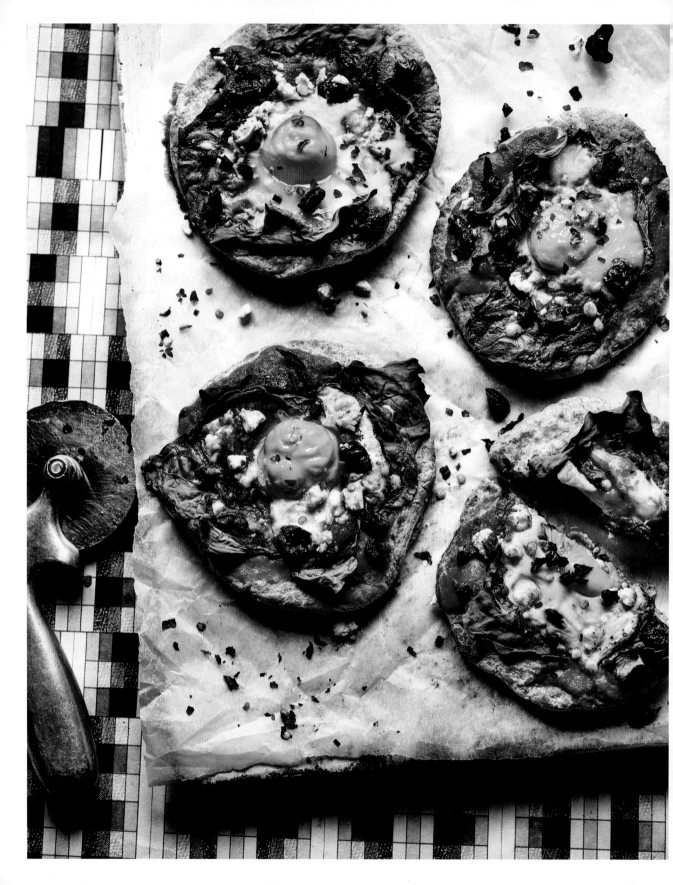

IT'S A PIZZA PITTA #CHEATDAY #FAKEAWAY #MEATFREEMONDAY

MAKES 2

It's a pizza, but not quite as you know it – a cross-cultural version which uses pitta bread for ease. Yes, it's your cheat day, so you can order a pizza if you fancy it, but I genuinely love these homemade versions. They are fun and easy to make, plus they arrive in my mouth faster than a takeaway does. Result. Feel free to play around with your favourite toppings – if you want extra protein, tuna goes well. They are tried and tested on my little cousins, so if you have kids, these have got the thumbs up… although you may have the plate returned with the olives rejected!

Preheat the oven to 190°C (375°F), Gas Mark 5.

Spread a layer of passata over each pitta, then sprinkle over the oregano and chilli flakes. Now arrange a border of overlapping spinach leaves around the edges of each bread, leaving a small gap in the centre.

Sprinkle the olives over the breads, then crack 1 egg into the gap left in the centre of each bread. Scatter over the crumbled feta.

Lay the pizza breads on a baking tray and bake for 15–20 minutes, until the egg whites are set.

3 tablespoons passata (a version with basil, if possible)
2 wholemeal or seeded pitta breads (I like to use circular ones for a mini pizza look)
½ teaspoon dried oregano
2 small pinches of chilli flakes
handful of spinach leaves
1 tablespoon black olives, chopped
2 eggs
a little feta cheese, crumbled

TIP:

These can be enjoyed cold for a post-workout lunch or breakfast, so prepare more than you need and you won't need to worry about cooking the next day.

SPEEDY BLACK FOREST BITES
#CHEATDAY

MAKES 6

These little mounds of cherry chocolate can help you avoid eating an entire chocolate bar in one sitting… and they contain cherries, which are antioxidant central. Happy days. Or use raspberries if you prefer. Both are made to be encased in rich chocolate, if you ask me.

Lay the cherry halves on a sheet of baking paper and freeze for 20 minutes.

Once the cherries are just about or almost frozen, melt the chocolate in a heatproof bowl set over a pan of simmering water.

Lay a fresh sheet of baking paper on a baking sheet. Arrange the cherries on the paper in little mounds of 4-5 cherry halves. Sprinkle each pile with some chopped macadamia nuts.

Pour roughly 1½ tablespoons melted chocolate over each mound. The chocolate will trickle down the sides of the mounds, but the cherries will still remain visible in places.

Freeze on the sheet for another 20 minutes, until the chocolate has set hard, then transfer to a sealed plastic container and freeze, ready for when you fancy them.

```
200g (7oz) cherries, halved
    and pitted
100g (3½oz) dark chocolate
    (minimum 70 per cent cocoa
    solids)
handful of macadamia nuts,
    chopped
```

TIP:

This should be where I tell you how long these bites last, but I have no idea because they are always gone by the end of my cheat day and I usually have my head in that box within an hour of putting it in the freezer! Instead, I will tell you that if you use raspberries instead of cherries, chopped blanched almonds work well in place of the macadamia nuts.

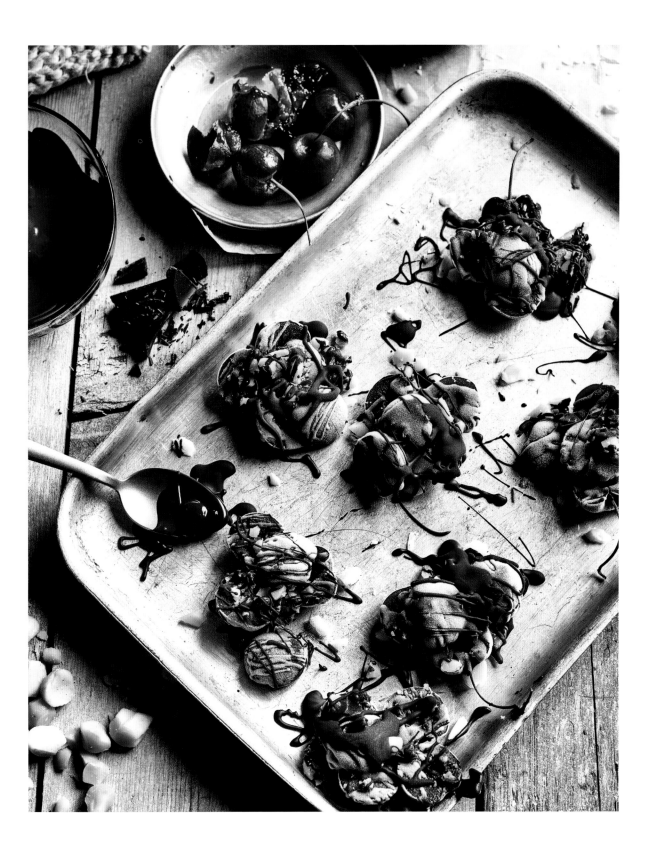

BOUNTY SEA SALT BOMBS #CHEATDAY   MAKES 22–24

I serve these up as energy balls on my fitness retreats, without
the cocoa, and they are probably our most requested recipe. I
can't take credit for them unfortunately – the recipe is a Mrs PMA
special. It's in the cheat day section because we can have these in
the house only on a Sunday as I just can't resist them. I swear she
puts some secret addictive ingredient in them! Make a batch and
you'll see what I mean.

Place all the ingredients into a food processor and pulse until the mixture sticks
together when you pinch it and the cashews and dates are finely chopped. Add
more coconut oil if needed. Roll the mixture into balls.

Spread some desiccated coconut on a plate. Mix some more desiccated
coconut with a little cocoa powder in a bowl. Roll half the balls in one mixture,
and half in the other.

Transfer the balls to an airtight container and store in the refrigerator. They will
keep for about a week (so, 2 cheat days) if you don't finish them in one go.

55g (2oz) unsalted cashews
9 Medjool dates, pitted
¼ teaspoon ground sweet
    cinnamon
¼ teaspoon vanilla extract
140g (5oz) desiccated coconut,
    plus extra for rolling
large pinch of fine sea salt
2½ teaspoons dark cocoa powder,
    plus extra for rolling
2½ tablespoons coconut oil,
    plus extra as required

COOKIES AND MILK #CHEATDAY

Can you beat warm, soft cookies straight from the oven? I use coconut sugar in these, which is slightly better for us than regular sugar. These cookies are so quick and easy to make, you can whiz some up in the time it takes to go to the shops and buy a packet filled with additives and preservatives. Eat them while they are still chewy and gooey from the oven and don't forget a cold glass of milk for the full cheat day experience.

Preheat the oven to 180°C (350°F), Gas Mark 4. Line a baking sheet with kitchen foil and grease it lightly with spray oil.

Mix the sugar and melted coconut oil in a large bowl. I use the back of the spoon to grind the granules up slightly and mix them into the oil. Spend about a minute on this stage, then add the egg yolk, vanilla extract, bicarbonate of soda and the dark cocoa powder, if using, and mix until thoroughly combined.

Mix in the flour – this takes time, but be patient. Once it reaches the point when it is almost mixed but a little "bitty", use your hands to bring the dough together. If needed, you can add an extra ¼–½ teaspoon melted coconut oil if the mixture is too dry and still crumbly. You should end up with a nice smooth cookie dough.

Roll the dough into a ball with your hands, then divide it into 6 even portions. Roll each of these into a ball in your hands, rolling a few of the chocolate chips into the balls, and also the blanched hazelnut halves, if using.

Arrange the balls on the prepared baking sheet with plenty of space between them to allow the cookies to expand as they cook. Squish down the balls into circles, but don't completely flatten them. Top with the remaining dark chocolate chips.

Bake at the centre of the oven for 10 minutes, until dry on top and slightly cracked.

Leave to cool slightly on the baking sheet for a few minutes, until firm enough to transfer onto a wire rack. Leave on the wire rack to cool completely – or attack them while they are still warm!

spray oil, for greasing

55g (2oz) coconut sugar

25g (1oz) coconut oil, melted, plus extra as required

1 egg yolk

1 teaspoon vanilla extract

½ teaspoon bicarbonate of soda

1 teaspoon dark cocoa powder (optional)

55g (2oz) plain wholemeal flour

handful of dark chocolate chips

handful of halved blanched hazelnuts (optional)

TIP:

The cookies may seem uncooked when you take them out of the oven because they will still be very soft, but they continue to cook and harden outside of the oven, until you have crunchy cookies. In my opinion, they are at their best about 10 minutes after cooking, when they are still warm, soft and chewy.

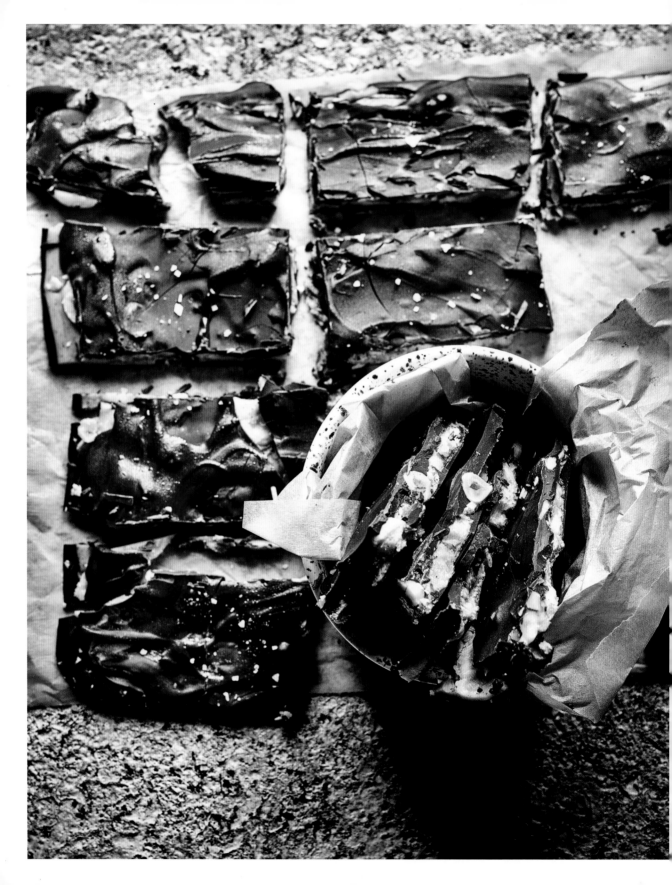

CHOCONUT BANANA SLAB
#CHEATDAY

I don't even need to introduce this one because the ingredients do all the talking. Chocolate, banana, peanut butter, toasted hazelnuts. *mic drop*

Melt 100g (3½oz) of the dark chocolate in a heatproof bowl set over a pan of simmering water. Meanwhile, melt the peanut butter in a cup in the microwave for a few seconds. (If you don't have a microwave, melt it in a saucepan set over a low heat, whisking it as it becomes liquid.)

Lay a sheet of baking paper on a baking sheet. Pour the melted chocolate onto the paper, and use the back of a spoon to smooth it out into a rectangular shape measuring roughly 25 x 15cm (10 x 6 inches).

Drizzle the melted peanut butter over the chocolate, then lay the banana slices on top so they are fairly close but not touching. Scatter over the chopped hazelnuts. Transfer the tray to the freezer and chill for 10–15 minutes.

Melt the remaining chocolate as before, then spoon it over the frozen slab to cover the bananas and all the way to the edges of the slab to seal it all together.

Freeze for a further 20 minutes, then remove the baking paper from the tray. Lay the slab on a chopping board and quickly slice it with a sharp knife into 9–12 squares. Place them in a sealable plastic container or freezer bag and store in the freezer until you fancy a nibble.

300g (10½oz) dark chocolate (minimum 70 per cent cocoa solids)

3 tablespoons smooth peanut butter

1 banana, cut into 3mm (1/8 inch) slices

2 tablespoons chopped toasted hazelnuts

TIP:

Adding a little sprinkle of fine sea salt when you add the hazelnuts is pretty magical!

ALMOND BUTTER BANANA BREAD MUFFINS #CHEATDAY

MAKES 10

Creating the recipe for these banana bread muffins was one of those happy accidents you sometimes have in the kitchen. I was trying to follow a recipe and realised I had none of the right ingredients, so threw in a few different things and hoped for the best. By some miracle, something came out that wasn't just edible, but delicious. It was supposed to be a banana bread loaf because that's one of my favourite indulgences, but I didn't have a tin, so the banana bread muffins were born. And now I'm too scared to change the recipe in case it goes wrong, so they are here to stay.

Preheat the oven to 180°C (350°F), Gas Mark 4. Grease a 12-hole muffin tin.

Put the muffin ingredients into a blender and blend until smooth.

Pour the mixture into 10 of the holes in the prepared muffin tin, filling each hole about three-quarters full so there is space for the muffins to rise. At this point you can add your chosen toppings. I like chopped pecans with banana slices on some, and chocolate chips with banana on the rest. Alternatively, bake them plain and top after baking (*see* tip).

Bake for 15–17 minutes, until cooked through. Leave to cool in the muffin tin.

spray oil or coconut oil,
  for greasing
3 bananas (the riper the better)
2 eggs
175g (6oz) rolled oats
5 Medjool dates, pitted
2 tablespoons almond butter
1 teaspoon ground sweet cinnamon
1 teaspoon bicarbonate of soda
1 tablespoon maple syrup

Optional toppings:
½ banana, sliced
3–4 tablespoons roughly chopped
  pecan nuts
3 tablespoons smooth peanut
  butter, melted
3–4 tablespoons dark chocolate
  chips

TIP:

If you don't top the muffins before baking, melted peanut butter is a dreamy post-baking topping. Melt 3 tablespoons smooth peanut butter in the microwave for a few seconds, then rub it over the muffin tops. Sprinkle over 3–4 tablespoons chopped pecans to finish. Alternatively, mix 1½ tablespoons cream cheese, 1 tablespoon Greek yogurt and 1 teaspoon maple syrup in a bowl until smooth. Spread it over the plain muffins, then top with 3–4 tablespoons chopped pecans and a sprinkling of sweet cinnamon. Refrigerate your peanut butter and cream cheese versions so the topping can set.

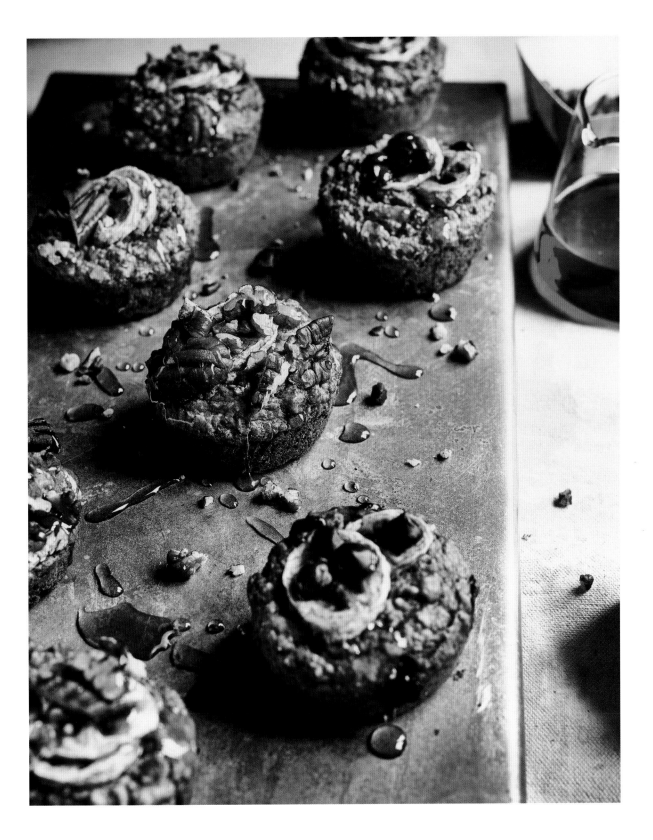

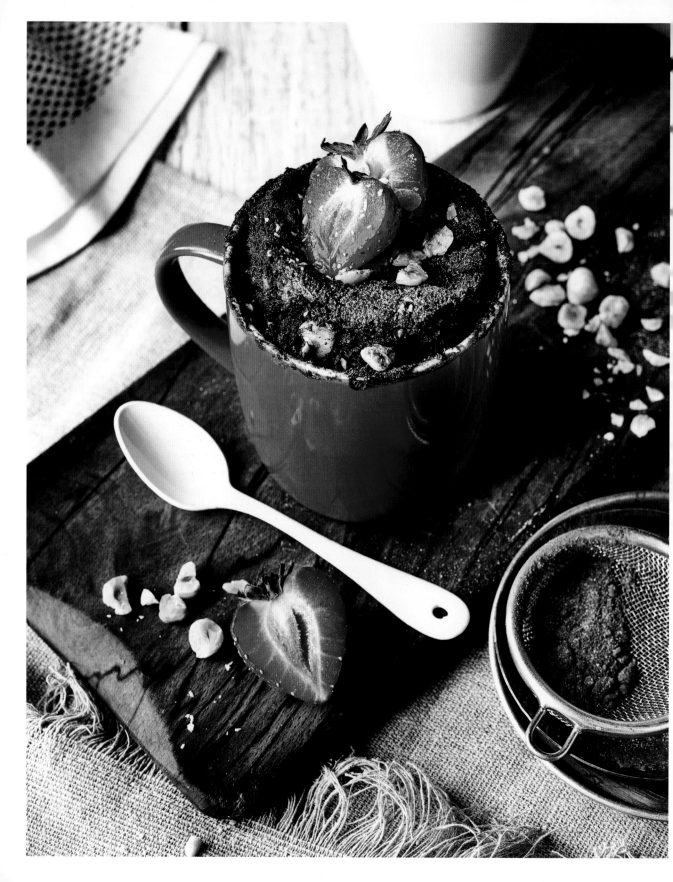

CHOCOLATE ESPRESSO CUPCAKE #CHEATDAY

Attention! This is a gooey chocolate cake that you can prepare and cook in no more than three minutes. (You're welcome.) A small amount of coffee gives it a nice rich flavour, while the sweetness of the banana means you can keep the sugar content relatively low. No electric whisks, no blenders, no ovens, no cake tins, no fuss. (Like I said guys, you're welcome!)

Combine the dry ingredients in a bowl. Whisk together the wet ingredients in a jug. Slowly add the wet ingredients to the bowl and stir until thoroughly mixed.

Pour the mixture into a large mug or cup, then microwave for 60–80 seconds, depending on the strength of your microwave. The cake should rise and have a sponge-like cakey top with pockets of melted goodness inside.

Decorate with the strawberry and extra hazelnuts.

1 tablespoon plain wholemeal flour
1 tablespoon dark cocoa powder
½ tablespoon coconut sugar
½ teaspoon bicarbonate of soda
½ teaspoon instant coffee granules
10 whole blanched hazelnuts, plus extra to decorate
1½ teaspoons dark chocolate chips
½ ripe banana (overripe is even better)
2½ tablespoons almond milk
1 tablespoon smooth peanut butter
1 egg yolk
1 strawberry, halved, to decorate

TIP:

Pour a little bit of cream into the middle if you want to take Cheat Day up a notch.

CONCLUSION

By now, it should be very clear to you just how close a link there is between body and mind. If you want to succeed in your training goals, it is imperative that, going forward, you continue to train both body and mind - if you neglect one, the other will suffer. In this book, I give you the tools you need to really make a go of this task.

If you've always wanted to be fitter, or you've always dreamed of being stronger, there's no reason why you can't be. Take this opportunity to start again and finally nail those goals. My 14-day plan gives you the perfect reset, so you move forward from a fresh slate and work toward achieving a stronger, fitter, healthier version of you. This is you versus you now, and you've got to fight to make sure the right side of you wins.

You don't need to overhaul your life - these are not huge adjustments we're talking about. But the changes you make, if you stick with them, will create life-improving results. Take everything you've learned in this book and apply it to your everyday life until it becomes as natural as brushing your teeth. If you find yourself slipping back into old habits, don't worry. It's not the end of the world. Just re-focus your energy and start the plan again from day one. You will get there eventually and that's all that matters.

PMA - keeping a positive mental attitude - will absolutely change your life for the better, but I recognize that for some people it comes easier than it does for others. That's okay. It is okay for things to be hard. What isn't okay is to give up when things get tough. You deserve better than that. Once you've nailed that emotional fitness and started to believe in what's possible, I can assure you the rest will follow and you will never look back. Success is 100 per cent down to body and 100 per cent down to mind. The two work in perfect harmony to create a circle that just keeps on giving.

The most important thing to remember in all of this is it should be fun. Exercise can and should be enjoyable, I promise! Sometimes you just need to stick with it and ride the waves until you reach the fun, smoother sailing part.

Throughout this process, never forget that you are doing this for you, nobody else. You have your own goals and your own demons and you can expect to have your own successes and failures along the way. None of us are built the same, and that's what makes us so awesome, so if the person next to you is slimmer, more toned, stronger, fitter or faster - who cares?! That is no reason to give up.

If you can always say that you are giving it your best and your 100 per cent then you can hold your head up high and tell yourself that you are one seriously kickass individual. Yes, you are striving to be the best version of yourself, but you should still love yourself for who you are right now because a little bit of love goes a long way in the PMA game. Self-loathing and never feeling good enough aren't motivators, they are the ball and chain which make you feel like you do not deserve more. Not on my watch!

The final piece of advice I would like you to remember is this - always remember to celebrate how far you have come and don't fret about how far you have left to go. This isn't a journey with an end point, it's a totally new lifestyle for you to embrace forever, so stop panicking that the finish line is too far in the distance for you to see. There is no finish line. There is just your start line and, the better you get, the further away that start lines gets.

Now look in the mirror and tell yourself you've got this, because there's no time for tomorrows. The new, better you starts right here, right now. Good luck, and welcome to the #PMA family.

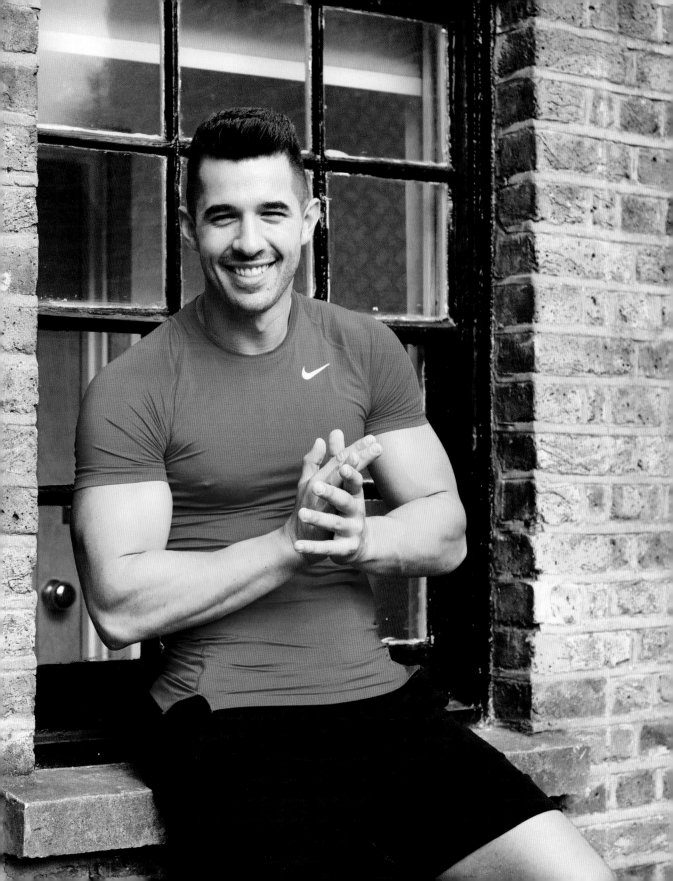

INDEX

I WOULD LIKE TO DEDICATE THIS BOOK TO ALL MY CLIENTS AND ONLINE FOLLOWERS WHO SHOW ME NOTHING BUT LOVE AND SUPPORT. YOU BLOW ME AWAY EVERY DAY WITH YOUR LOVELY MESSAGES. YOU ARE THE PEOPLE WHO INSPIRE ME TO DO EVERYTHING IN MY POWER TO MAKE SURE THE MESSAGE OF PMA CONTINUES TO SPREAD FAR AND WIDE. WITHOUT YOU ALL, THERE WOULD BE NO BOOK AT ALL. SO THANK YOU.

ACKNOWLEDGEMENTS

Firstly, I'd like to say a huge thank you to everybody at Barry's Bootcamp for believing in me and giving me the opportunity to become the trainer that I am today. You changed my life, opening up a world of opportunities I could never have dreamed of. You are all my family and I love you dearly.

Big thanks also to my Nike crew who have sent me around the world with my training and allowed me to expand my trainer collection beyond belief. You took me under your wing and helped shape me as a man and a trainer, and I hope I can pass on everything you taught me to the future Nike generations for years to come.

Shout out to my homegirl Ellie Goulding. You have supported me from the start and I am privileged to have worked with you for so long. My Meatfree Monday recipes are dedicated to you and I hope they play even the smallest part in making a difference.

Another person who has supported me with no agenda other than the fact he's an amazing guy is Joe Wicks AKA The Body Coach. You are an inspiration to millions around the world, me included. You have changed the face of fitness and I will always be grateful for the opportunities you have thrown my way.

I'd also like to thank my superstar team at Becca Barr Management. Without you, I would never have dreamed of writing this book. Thank you for believing in me and being patient when I'm lifting s instead of adulting and responding to emails.

It goes without saying that the whole team at Octopus deserve a big up. You are all incredible and have helped

make the impossible possible. I am sorry for disturbing you all with my very loud voice in all of our meetings – the office isn't my natural habitat! Thanks also to the insanely talented photographers Kris Kirkham and Philip Haynes, as well as my man crush/hero/videographer Barnaby Riggs, who has been with me from the start.

Props to my friends and the training community in and around London (you know who you are) who train with me, sweat with me, hold cameras for me without complaining and push me constantly. I learn something new from you every day.

To everyone that has contributed to this book, by sending in testimonials and PMA pose photos, or who follow me online, thank you. I can never express what an impact you have all had on my life.

Now to get soppy. To my family, thank you for raising me to believe I can achieve anything I set my mind to. You instilled a positive mental attitude in me from birth and I hope that one day, when I raise my own family, I can pass on even a fraction of the life lessons you taught me. I love you all to the moon and back.

And finally, I would like to thank my wife, Mrs PMA. You are the most incredibly talented woman and I am blessed to have you in my life. Quite simply, this book would not have been written had it not been for your tireless efforts in helping to make it happen. You make me a better man and everything I do, every early morning alarm and every late night, is for you. You are my world and there is nobody else I'd rather have with me on this ride. I love you.